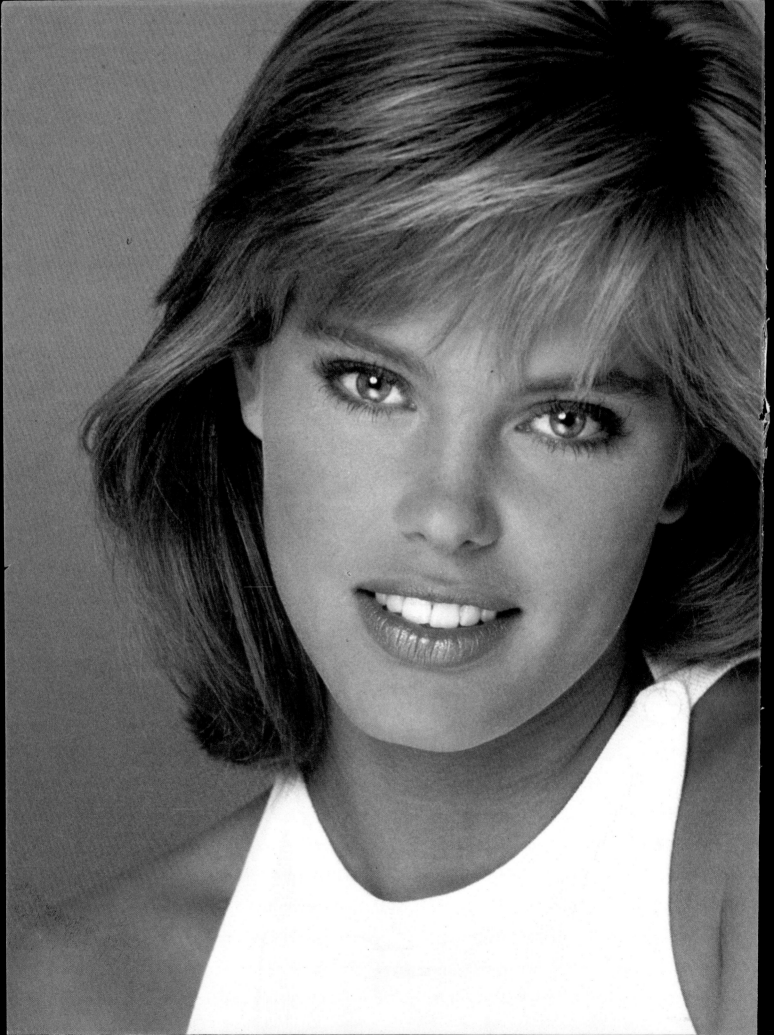

The Ford Models' Crash Course in Looking Great

❧

EILEEN FORD

and JOAN R. HEILMAN

SPECIAL PHOTOGRAPHS BY HARRISON GOULD

SIMON AND SCHUSTER   *NEW YORK*

Renée Simonsen

Published by Simon and Schuster
A Division of Simon & Schuster, Inc.
Simon & Schuster Building
Rockefeller Center
1230 Avenue of the Americas
New York, New York 10020
SIMON AND SCHUSTER and colophon are registered trademarks of
Simon & Schuster, Inc.

Designed by Irving Perkins Associates

Manufactured in Spain by Novograph, S.A., Madrid

1   2   3   4   5   6   7   8   9   10

Library of Congress Cataloging in Publication Data

Ford, Eileen.
    The Ford models' crash course in looking great.

    1. Beauty, Personal. 2. Skin—Care and hygiene.
3. Cosmetics. 4. Hairdressing. 5. Reducing diets—
Menus. 6. Reducing exercises. I. Heilman, Joan Rattner.
II. Title.

RA778.F7197   1985   646.7′042   84-29796
ISBN: 0-671-49961-0

PHOTO CREDITS

David Bailey: p. 253 (courtesy *Vogue,* copyright 1967 by the Condé Nast Publications, Inc.).

Dick Ballerian: pp. 73, 116, 246 (courtesy *Harper's Bazaar,* copyright 1982 by the Hearst Corporation); p. 128 (courtesy Harper's Bazaar, copyright 1983 by the Hearst Corporation).

Blanch: pp. 22, 66, 138 (courtesy *Vogue,* copyright 1982 by the Condé Nast Publications, Inc.).

Eric Boman: pp. 2, 243 (courtesy *Self,* copyright 1983 by the Condé Nast Publications, Inc.).

Alex Chatelain: p. 130 (courtesy *Vogue,* copyright 1979 by the Condé Nast Publications, Inc.).

Patrick Demarchelier: pp. 14, 19 (bottom), (courtesy *Harper's Bazaar,* copyright 1984 by the Hearst Corporation); p. 35 (courtesy *Self,* copyright 1984 by the Condé Nast Publications, Inc.).

Arthur Elgort: pp. 19 (top), 86 (courtesy *Vogue,* copyright 1981 by the Condé Nast Publications, Inc.); p. 48 (courtesy *Vogue,* copyright 1978 by the Condé Nast Publications, Inc.); pp. 92 (both), 98, 99 (bottom), 114 (courtesy *Vogue,* copyright 1979 by the Condé Nast Publications, Inc.); p. 133 (courtesy *Vogue,* copyright 1982 by the Condé Nast Publications, Inc.).

Jo Francki: pp. 29, 99 (top), (courtesy *Vogue,* copyright 1980 by the Condé Nast Publications, Inc.).

Gerard Gentil: p. 141 (left).

Mark Glasser: p. 119.

Marco Glaviano: pp. 40, 82 (courtesy *Vogue,* copyright 1981 by the Condé Nast Publications, Inc.).

Les Goldberg: pp. 47, 254 (courtesy *France Harper's Bazaar,* copyright 1984 by the Hearst Corporation).

Harrison Gould: pp. 18, 26 (both), 27 (both), 28 (both), 32, 34, 37, 38, 56, 59, 60, 70, 81, 89, 90, 93–97 (all), 102 (both), 120–23 (all), 141 (right), 144, 147, 150, 154, 157, 160, 163, 184, 188–200 (all), 202–7 (all), 208–15 (all), 217, 219–21 (all), 223–31 (all), 232, 234–38 (all).

Tom Hooper: p. 106 for Coty.

Horst: p. 250 (courtesy *Vogue,* copyright 1954 by the Condé Nast Publications, Inc.).

Frank Horvat: p. 167 (courtesy *Glamour,* copyright 1983 by the Condé Nast Publications, Inc.).

Paul Lange: p. 145 (courtesy *Glamour,* copyright 1983 by the Condé Nast Publications, Inc.).

Jacques Malignon: pp. 6, 67 (courtesy *Harper's Bazaar,* copyright 1982 by the Hearst Corporation); pp. 43, 57, 170, 177 (courtesy *Harper's Bazaar,* copyright 1984 by the Hearst Corporation).

Stan Malinowski: pp. 24, 68, 125 (courtesy *Harper's Bazaar,* copyright 1984 by the Hearst Corporation), 180, 222.

Duane Michals: p. 30 (courtesy *Vogue,* copyright 1975 by the Condé Nast Publications, Inc.).

Gordon Munro: p. 111.

Penn: pp. 107 (courtesy *Vogue,* copyright 1982 by the Condé Nast Publications, Inc.), 247 (courtesy *Vogue,* copyright 1949 by the Condé Nast Publications, Inc.).

Rico Puhlmann: pp. 20 (both), 77, 175, 216, 252 (courtesy *Harper's Bazaar,* copyright 1984 by the Hearst Corporation); pp. 61, 201, 233 (courtesy *Harper's Bazaar,* copyright 1983 by the Hearst Corporation).

Mike Reinhardt: p. 10 (courtesy *Harper's Bazaar,* copyright 1983 by the Hearst Corporation).

Al Rubin: p. 55.

Skrebneski: pp. 44, 64 (for Estee Lauder).

Bert Stern: p. 249 (courtesy *Vogue,* copyright 1970 by the Condé Nast Publications, Inc.).

Photos pp. 244, 255 for Revlon. Page 245 courtesy *Vogue,* copyright 1952 by the Condé Nast Publications, Inc. Page 248 courtesy the Condé Nast Publications, Inc.

ALSO BY EILEEN FORD

Eileen Ford's Beauty Now and Forever
A More Beautiful You in 21 Days
Secrets of the Model's World
Eileen Ford's Book of Model Beauty

ACKNOWLEDGMENTS

There are many thanks due to many people who helped with this book. Thanks, of course, to all the Ford models who contributed their beauty tips and wisdom. To Harrison Gould, who gave his time and talent to producing the photographs that needed to be shot specially for the book. To *Harper's Bazaar* and the Condé Nast magazines—*Vogue*, *Glamour*, and *Self*—which were more than generous in allowing us to use photographs of Ford models that have appeared on their pages. To Betty Klarnet and Myrna Borsuk at *Harper's Bazaar* and Cynthia Cathcart at Condé Nast for their help in gathering them. To Lacey Ford and her assistant Susan Geer, who prepared the exercises. To Nancy Noonan, who, in addition to her arduous duties as head of Ford Promotion, coordinated the acquisition of the artwork. To Marion Smith who served as liaison with the models.

We are especially grateful to the world-famous photographers who gave permission to use their published and unpublished work: David Bailey, Dick Ballerian, Andrea Blanch, Eric Boman, Alex Chatelain, Patrick Demarchelier, Arthur Elgort, Jo Francki, Gerard Gentil, Mark Glasser, Marco Glaviano, Les Goldberg, Tom Hooper, Horst, Frank Horvat, Paul Lange, Jacques Malignon, Stan Malinowski, Duane Michals, Gordon Munro, Penn, Rico Puhlmann, Mike Reinhardt, Al Rubin, Skrebneski, Bert Stern.

I would like to thank Joan Heilman for doing the research, interviewing the models and pushing all of us until the job was complete.

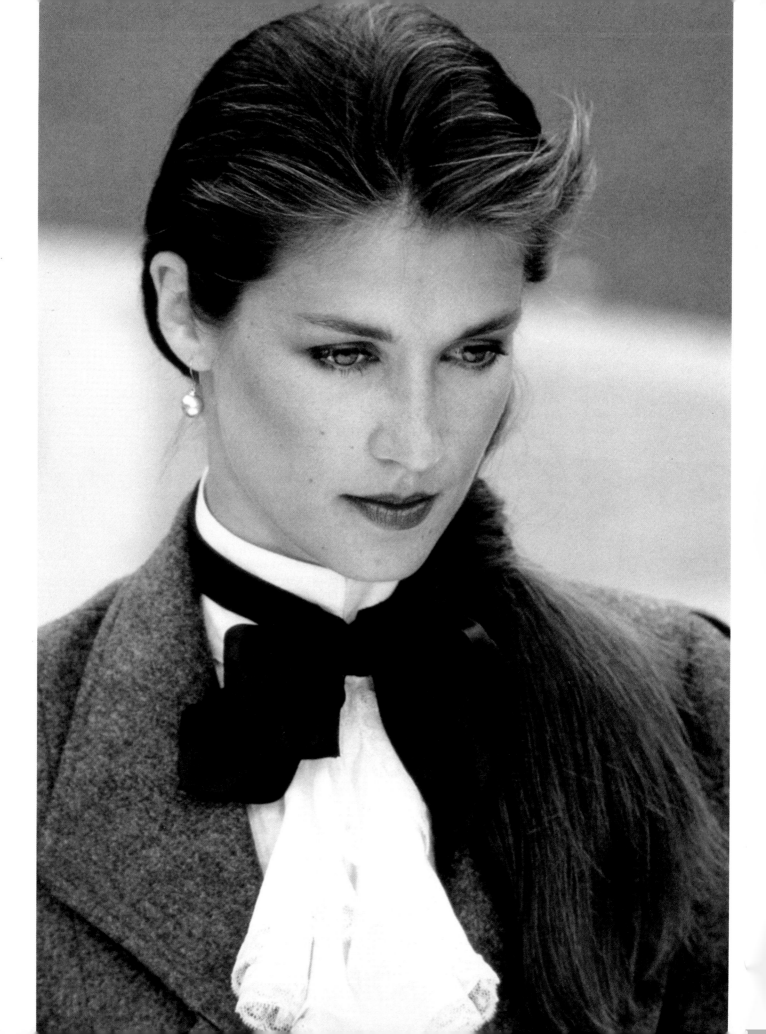

CONTENTS

Clotilde

The Ford Models' Crash Course in Looking Great

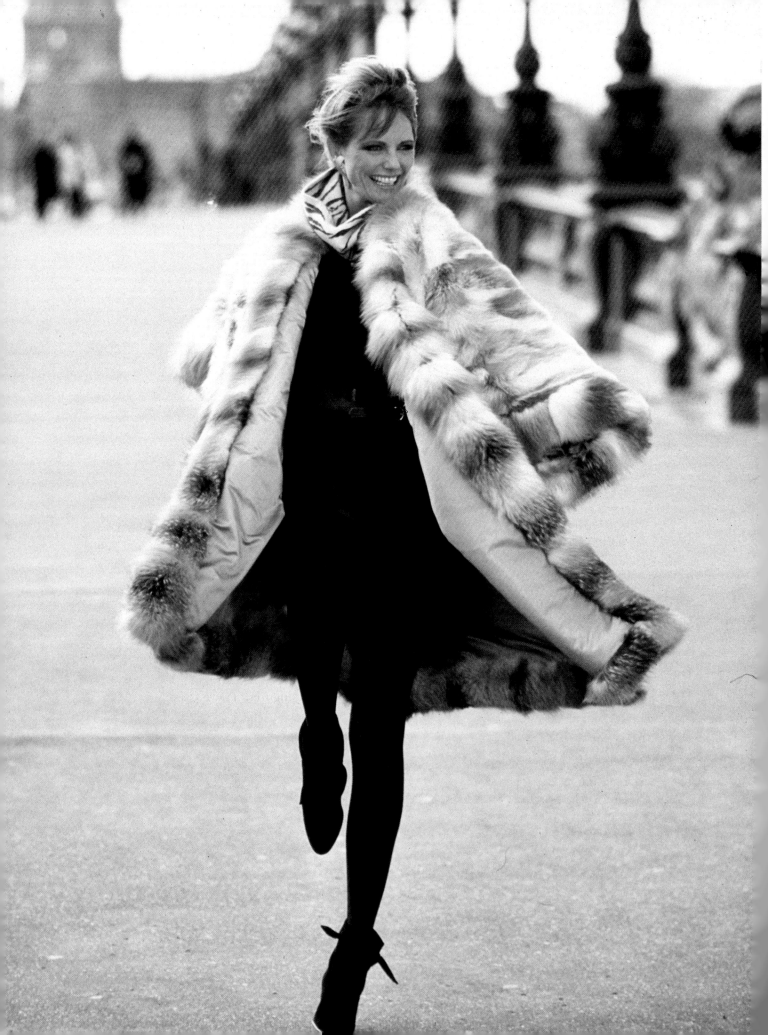

HOW YOU CAN LOOK LIKE A MODEL

As you know, the name of this book is *The Ford Models' Crash Course in Looking Great*, a very descriptive title. This book is designed to give you, the reader, the way to redesign your looks—and your lifestyle—in a hurry. Ford models share with you their trade secrets, the tricks they have learned from makeup artists, invented themselves, or exchanged with one another.

Models are professional beauties. In a sense, they are the super salespeople of the cosmetics, fashion, fragrance and hair-products industries. Their faces and figures show other women what is the latest and the best in these worlds. Without the help of a great model working with a great photographer, I sincerely doubt these businesses would have developed the way they have. The money that models make for posing in these ads is well known. Contracts for exclusivity with a product or line of clothing can run into hundreds of thousands of dollars, even into the millions. Why are models so well paid? Great models are responsible for great sales figures. There is no one else in the world who can sell their products so well.

The livelihoods of professional beauties such as models depend on their good looks. Their health, their skin, their bodies, their makeup and their hair, even their hands and feet, are their sales tools and they require the same care an artist gives his brushes. Diet, exercise and makeup techniques are their lives. Our models have very generously opened their whole bag of tricks for you to explore. They have shared with you their knowledge of how to make yourself look great.

"Crash course" implies speedy and that is what I meant it to do. This book is a fast, authoritative beauty plan tailored for you by the world's beauty authorities, the Ford models; and by me, since I have made up what I think are two wonderful diets. One diet is for those who like to cook, the other for those who can't or won't.

If you read carefully and follow these tips, there is no reason why you too should not look like a model beauty in very little time. None of us is born perfect. Everyone can use help and help is here; all you have to do is read, learn and practice to crash through to beauty.

Cheryl Tiegs

You have your own beauty potential, and even if you're not planning a modeling career, you can make the best of what you've got. The self-confidence that follows, and the esteem of others, will brighten your life. The future will be sunnier because you will know that your "You Potential" has been developed and you will thrive on it.

WHO THE FORDS ARE

It all started in October, 1946, when I was young, married, and pregnant, and offered to handle the phone calls of two friends who were models, because we needed the money. Soon there were four more models asking for my help in keeping track of their bookings. My husband, Jerry, who had been a football player at Notre Dame and an ensign in the Navy during World War II and was now working for my father, sold our car to pay the rent on a small office on New York's Second Avenue, and we started a business. At the end of a year, we had acquired 36 models, and by 1948 we had seven telephones and were grossing a quarter of a million dollars a year—big money in those days. Today we run a $30-million-a-year business, the largest and the best-known model agency in the world.

Three of our four children work with us, and we all have well-defined roles. I manage the models. Jerry runs the business. Billy is in charge of promotion and the search for new models. Katie is financial director and Lacey runs the special projects, including the "Face of the '80s," an annual international model search.

WHO THE MODELS ARE

- The most successful models today are not supersophisticated, haughty, ethereal, sweetly pretty, or remote as they once were. They have a natural, healthy glow, a friendly open look, as well as elegance and femininity.

- Currently, the majority of our best models are Americans. Even among those working in Europe, about 65 percent are from the U.S. For some reason, our best sources are northern Florida, California, Texas and Ohio. And, of course, New York, which is a magnet for attractive, ambitious young girls.

- Models today are much taller than they used to be. The typical model about ten years ago was five feet seven inches tall. Now we look for girls who are at least five-eight and some are five-eleven. Even a classic beauty who isn't the right height isn't accepted because the clothes, usually designers' samples made on tall showroom models, won't fit.

- Models last a long time today if they behave in a rational way and take good care of themselves. There are many more than you'd ever dream working right through their thirties and occasionally beyond. They have to start out very young, of course, but they last.

- Though there's little room in a heavily booked model's existence for more than work and beauty care and sleep, it is an exciting life. What could be more thrilling than having a pin stuck in you by Yves St. Laurent or Calvin Klein? What's more luxurious than being swathed in sable and covered with diamond and emerald jewels? Or more wonderful than flying off to work on location in Egypt, the Maldives or Paris?

- It's not easy to describe the qualifications we seek in a model, but to generalize, it's a face with character and strength as well as beauty, plus an ability to come alive for the camera. Physically, we look for girls with long legs and long necks. We like big, wide-set eyes, good skin, a firm, limber body, a straight nose, straight white teeth, a rather large sensuous mouth, and high cheekbones. Obviously, we don't find many girls who have the whole combination so we look for as many of those characteristics as we can put together.

- Even the most beautiful model looks better with the right makeup and hair. They all need help, just like you and me.

Now let's get on to more important matters—how you can reach your own beauty potential. Make use of the trade secrets of the Ford models. Follow their advice, and you, too, can have it all for yourself. I promise you, because I have seen it happen. Remember, there's not one trick the models use that you can't adopt for yourself to bring out your own individual beauty. Take the seven classes in the Ford Models' Crash Course in Looking Great and you'll see.

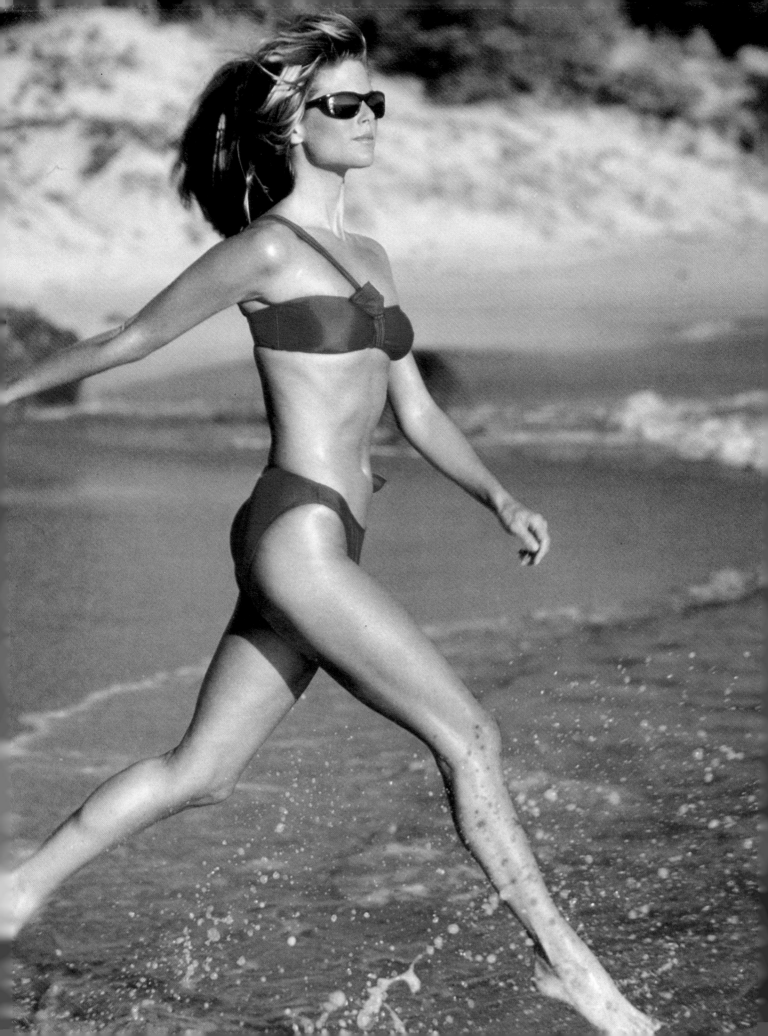

HOW TO HAVE SUPER SKIN

Every Ford model has a ritual, a private routine, for skin fitness, some more elaborate than others. I know girls who swear by yogurt inside and out, and some who mash avocados for a skin softener. I know models who buy nothing but the most expensive skin-care products sold in the best shops and salons, following the directions to the letter, and a growing number of others who insist on doing it *their* way, having found out by trial and error what works best to keep their skin glowing and clear. There are answers to every skin dilemma; it's simply a matter of discovering the right ones for you.

Many Ford models have achieved fame and fortune because of their exquisite skin. Jacki Adams, for example, is the only girl with whom Elizabeth Arden has ever signed an exclusive contract. Cheryl Tiegs and Christie Brinkley have been Cover Girl's image for many years. Lauren Hutton became world-famous as the face in the Revlon ads. Willow Bay's clean good looks have landed her a contract with Estée Lauder, Maura has a new four-year agreement with Clinique, Alda has signed with L'Oréal, and Nancy DeWeir is the girl you see in the Max Factor ads. Since their contracts are renewable, their futures depend on careful beauty practice, just what we're going to discuss in this chapter.

When girls first start out as Ford Models, makeup artists teach them how to make the most of themselves. Hairdressers give them tips on hair care. And skin-care specialists impress upon them the importance of taking care of the artist's canvas—their skin. And so do I! When a group of girls starts out together, I gather them in our conference room and give them my special talk. I explain what's expected of them as professional models, and I tell them what I've learned about caring for themselves inside and out, starting with their skin, which clearly reflects their lifestyle and daily habits.

YOUR FACE TELLS ON YOU

You cannot eat indiscriminately, drink a lot of alcohol or soda, smoke, stay out and dance all night, or experiment with drugs if you want beautiful

15

skin. Everything you do shows up on your face, now and later. I have been in this business for many years and I have seen hundreds and hundreds of models grow older. I can tell you which of them has consistently treated her body with respect, because it shows. It shows at the time, and it shows much more dramatically as the years go by. The women who have persisted in giving their skin careful attention are the ones who have continued to look fantastic. Jean Patchett, for example, probably the most photographed of any model of her time, is still a wonderful-looking woman. So is Lillian Marcuson, who was on more *Life* covers in the '50s than anyone except Dwight Eisenhower and is active to this day with our Classic Women division, and also Nan Rees, a vibrant "junior" and later a high-fashion model, who is an excellent example of what healthy habits will do for you.

BEWARE OF THE SUN!

The skin's enemy is the sun. You may look absolutely fabulous with a tan, but get a deep tan every year and by the time you are 40, your skin will show it. Even at 20, you'll have little lines that are yours for keeps. The effects of sun exposure are cumulative, can never be reversed once they've done their damage, and may lead to more serious problems than wrinkles.

Models today do not get deep tans. Most of them don't go out in the sun at all if they can help it, or they are very careful when they do. That's one way models have changed through the years—you don't see them baking on the beach anymore. The real problem arises when they work on location in the tropics. Kathryn Redding, for example, says you can always find her under a big hat in the shade. When she must emerge for a shot, she shields herself with an umbrella until the last moment.

Of course you cannot always position yourself under a tree, but you can protect your skin by using sunscreens that come in a range of strengths from very minimal protection up to a complete block of harmful rays. There are creams (best for dry skin), lotions (the choice for oily skin), gels. There are even moisturizers and foundations that contain sunscreens, though these usually have rather low SPF (Sun Protection Factor) ratings. The best products contain PABA or benzophenone (or both) which absorb ultraviolet rays. Never allow yourself to acquire more than a light tan, and get even that very gradually.

> **CHRISTIE BRINKLEY ON SUN:**
> *"Never sit with your face receiving direct sunlight without a sunscreen. The damage direct sun does to your face over time just isn't worth it. I collect hats, and I wear them or a sunscreen, and I find I get enough color in my face anyway."*

Apply sunscreen about half an hour before going out, and then reapply it every hour or so and after washing or swimming or working up a heavy sweat. Don't rub it in. Simply smooth it on in a rather thick layer.

Don't use baby oil or cocoa butter or other oils and greases to encourage tanning because they will make your skin fry.

Remember that even already-tanned skin needs protection, though perhaps a screen with a slightly lower SPF.

YOUR SKIN'S BEST FRIEND: WATER

More than anything else, your skin needs moisture. You must provide it both from within and without. Ford models drink lots of water. I hound them to drink six to eight big glasses every day, plus water-filled fruits and vegetables. It is not easy to get that much water into yourself until it becomes a habit, so I suggest you drink your water in the form that is the least objectionable to you. Tap water is fine, so is seltzer, mineral or spring water, water flavored with lemon juice, water perked up with juice, herbal tea, any way at all as long as you get it.

Maggie Fahy must float much of the time. "Nobody can believe the amount of water I drink," she insists. "Ice water. It cleans you out and plumps up your skin. I bet I drink two or three gallons a day." Donna Stia drinks hers without ice because for her it goes down more easily when it's not too cold. Cristina Ferrare likes it room temperature, too.

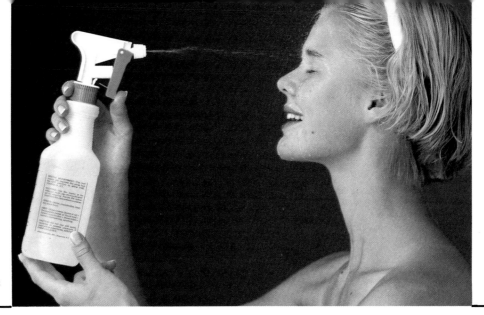

Anna Magnusson

That's the inside story. From the outside, moisturize. You must apply moisturizer constantly. Models are brainwashed never to go without it. Kelly LeBrock, who's one of our best English models and a film star too, keeps a tube of moisturizer in her car so she can smear it on her face every chance she gets.

Moisturizer doesn't add moisture. Instead, it seals in the water that is already in your skin so it doesn't evaporate into the atmosphere. Even very oily skin needs it on dry areas. Always apply it to skin that's been given a chance to absorb water first. Press a wet washcloth (make it *warm,* says Jennifer Berrington, to open your pores) to your face or splash your face with water, pat it almost off, then promptly smooth on a thin layer of moisturizer. After a bath or shower, apply it within one minute of stepping out of the tub. Juli Foster buys lots of different kinds of moisturizers and uses a different one every day so she'll get the benefits of all of them.

Avoid the dehydrators; these include alcohol, caffeine, diuretics (never take diuretics unless prescribed by your doctor for a specific medical condition—they are not cosmetics), and hot dry air.

A wise investment is a humidifier—or a few of them—for your living quarters, especially in winter. It compensates somewhat for central heating, high temperatures, dry climates, air conditioning.

Cristina Ferrare, a wonderful woman with a theory on everything, says she sleeps with the heat off and the humidifier on all year round. "If I'm traveling, I run a hot shower, and when the bathroom's steamy, I open the door." Maura, who's the woman you've been seeing in the Clinique ads for the last seven years and has signed on for another four, has a built-in steam room in her Malibu house on the beach and uses it a few times a week. In between, she takes care of her two babies, four horses and three dogs, and does her work. "Moisturizing is my most important beauty routine," she says.

If you have radiators, fill flat containers with water and put one on top of every radiator in the house. The trick is to keep them filled up. Plants help, too, if you remember to water them.

If you searched their big tote bags, you'd discover that an amazing number of models carry small spray bottles of natural spring water around with them. Whenever they feel dry, they take out the bottles and spray their faces with a fine mist. Kim Charlton, for example, has sprayed her face in the best of places.

Barbara Neumann

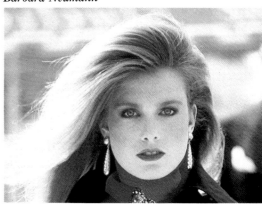

MODELS *are always taking high-flying jets to Tibet, or the Seychelles, or Paris, or maybe Hawaii. The dry air at high altitudes can be devastating to their skins. Barbara Neumann, for one, sprays her face and drinks a glass of water every hour during long flights to keep her skin moist.*

Christie Brinkley, like a lot of our other famous beauties, says water is her "secret weapon." She drinks it, breathes it (sleeps with a vaporizer in the room), sprays it on her face all day long.

Christie Brinkley

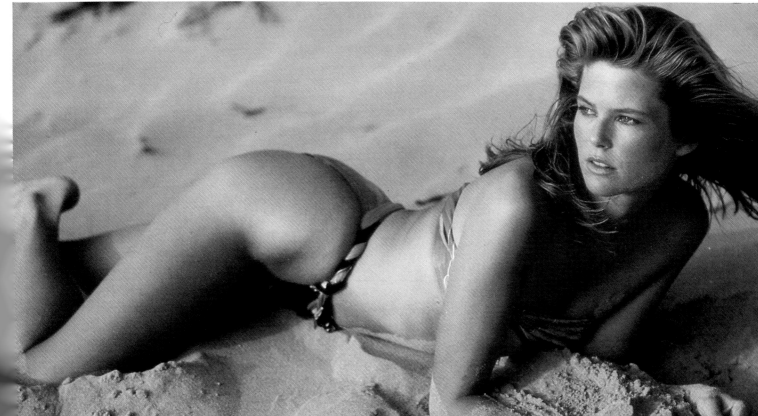

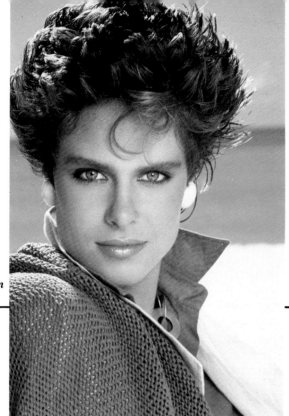

Kirsten Allen

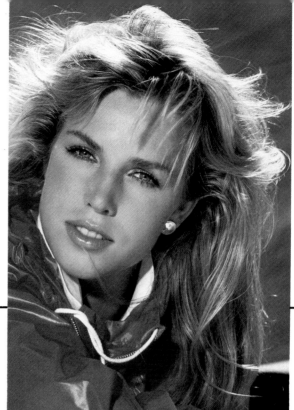

Anette Stai

DON'T BE TOO CLEAN

Baths and showers, especially hot, are extremely drying to your skin. Most dermatologists insist that Americans bathe too much and too long. If you have dry skin, two or three times a week is plenty in winter. Never use really hot water. Use a mild superfatted soap on your body (if your skin is dry, use the soap only on strategic areas). Don't stay in there and soak. Pat yourself dry. Then lubricate and/or moisturize.

Bath oil helps retain skin moisture, but only if you let the skin absorb the water first. Wait a while before adding the oil to the tub. A prominent dermatologist recommends swirling a cup of milk mixed with a capful of bath oil into the water. He says it's a most effective emollient.

ANY OIL WILL DO. *It doesn't matter whether you use expensive, exquisitely scented bath oil or simply pour some corn or sesame or even castor oil into your bath water. One of our "mature" models who wishes to remain anonymous always uses vitamin E oil in the tub, breaking open a couple of capsules. Nancy DeWeir likes almond oil, and Juli Foster prefers sesame.*

A really effective way to lubricate your body is to rub oil on *after* your shower. Carrie Miller—who decided on a whim to enter our "Face of the '80s" contest in 1983 and won it—steps out of the shower, applies baby oil all over her body, and then buffs it in with a towel.

DIET DON'TS

Healthy, resilient, glowing skin requires nourishing your body with the right foods and avoiding the wrong ones. Your diet should be full of fruits and vegetables, a few whole-grain foods, the leanest meats and fish, low-fat dairy products. Susan Hess, who's most concerned with healthy living habits, insists that everything that goes into your mouth turns up on your skin and I agree.

Foods to avoid are sweets and refined sugars, too much oil, alcohol, excessive iodine (in shellfish and iodized salt, for example), and bromide (in some antacids).

VITAMINS *help keep her skin in good condition in the winter, says Anette Stai, when she takes extra C and adds a vitamin B complex tablet to ward off outbreaks around the time of her period. Anette's the Norwegian girl who entered our international modeling contest in Monte Carlo a couple of years ago because she wanted to see Monte Carlo. She won, and now she's seen the world.*

THE SURPRISE INGREDIENT: EXERCISE

Exercise is essential for good skin. It stimulates circulation, bringing blood and nutrients to the surface. It gives you a glow and a healthy color you'll get no other way. Besides, perspiring is nature's way of moisturizing your epidermis.

Vibeke, whose incredible good looks after many years of modeling demonstrate the fact that it is *care* that counts, says, "I'm Danish and practical and see things very straightforward. I didn't do exercise much in Denmark,

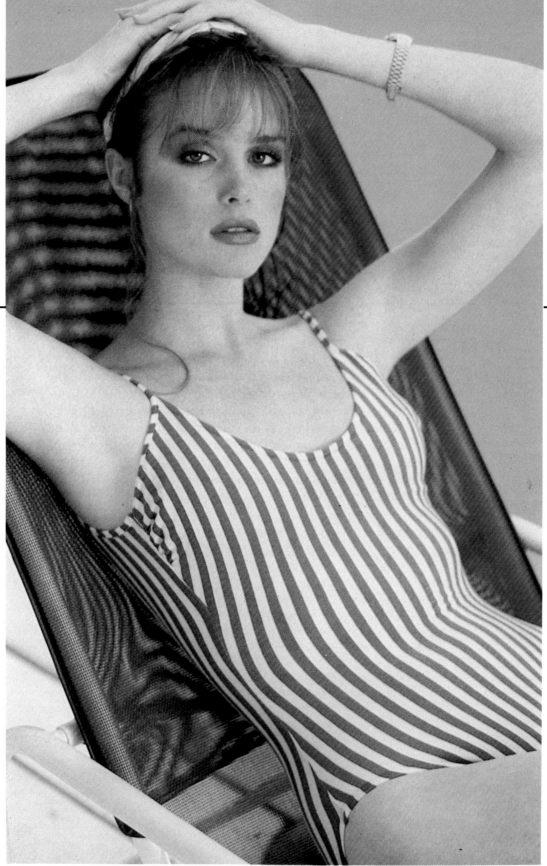

Jacki Adams

but now that I'm here and exercise all the time like the American girls, I see my skin is much more clear and healthy."

Willow Bay, an Estée Lauder spokeswoman (Karen Graham is another), says she *loves* to sweat. "It keeps your skin looking fresh. A good honest sweat is a natural cleanser."

SLEEPING IS SUPER

Even girls as young as most of our models can't get away with insufficient sleep. Jacki Adams says, "If I get really tired, I get dark circles under my eyes and my skin looks gray. You can't always camouflage that for the camera." Jacki, by the way, became one of our models when I made a quick trip to Florida to see her after a stranger sent snapshots. I knew immediately she would be a winner.

Cristina Ferrare, who's been modeling for a long time and still looks incredible, credits lots of sleep for her longevity at the top. She takes little catnaps, lying down, feet up, for 20 minutes or so whenever she needs a lift—or thinks her face does.

On the other hand, too much sleep is as bad as too little. It can make your eyes puffy and your face swollen. Find out how much sleep you need and get it. Christie Brinkley attributes her fresh good looks to the correct amount of sleep—"Less than six hours and I'm a wreck," she says. "More than seven and I'm groggy and look it."

> **SALADS, FRUITS AND LIQUIDS**
> *after about 7 p.m. make Rosemary McGrotha wake up in the morning with a puffy face. So she avoids them. But if she slips up, she wets a washcloth with ice water and presses it to her face. Rosemary, who's from Tallahassee, Fl., walked into Ford Models one day to try her luck. We signed her up on the spot. "In five minutes," she says, "I was a Ford model."*

OILY OR DRY?

The oil produced from the thousands of tiny sebaceous glands in your skin is your own natural moisturizer and lubricant. Whether your skin tends to be

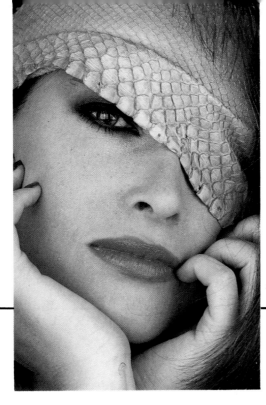

Rosemary McGrotha

normal, dry, or oily is a matter of heredity, and there's little you can do to change it. What you can do is help it maintain a healthy balance.

Most of us have "normal" skin, slightly oily down the center, and dryer along the sides and around the eyes. Dry skin doesn't make sufficient natural oil, so it tends to look dull and flaky. Oily skin, because it turns out excessive oil from those thousands of glands, is likely to look shiny and greasy and may tend to break out.

Oily skin, constantly lubricated and protected by the oil, ages much more slowly than the dry variety, so, if you've got it, be happy. You'll be getting compliments when you are 85. If you have excessively dry skin, you better replace what you're missing, or you won't!

THE NUMBER ONE RULE: KEEP IT CLEAN!

The most important ingredient of good skin care is cleansing. The first thing a model does when she gets home is to cleanse her face. She gets all that heavy makeup and accumulated dirt off as quickly and thoroughly as possible so her skin can breathe again. And I'll bet it's a very rare Ford model who doesn't walk around on her own time with little or no makeup on her face. That's a good idea for you, too. You may need some makeup for your everyday life and a lot more for special occasions, but when you're home or doing your own thing, let your skin have a rest. And never go to bed with your makeup on.

Soap or no soap? That is the question. There are no set rules. "Oils are good, soaps are good, creams are good, water is good—they are all good, but not for everyone," says one dermatologist. "Soap is irritating and harmful if you have very dry, sensitive skin, but there's nothing better than soap if you have plenty of oil." So, decide what kind of skin you have and proceed accordingly.

If you have sufficient oil in your skin and soap isn't too drying for you, use it. Renée Simonsen, the Danish girl who won our "Face of the '80s" contest in 1982, says she grew up on a soap-and-water routine, and she's sticking to it. Nancy DeWeir washes with soap. So does Erin Gray whose number one beauty secret, she says, is a clean face. Erin, star of a television series now, is proof that you can keep on looking wonderful if you treat yourself right. Carrie Miller uses unscented soap and carefully wipes off traces of eye makeup with moisturizer on a Q-tip.

If your skin is dry, perhaps the superfatted soaps will provide enough lubrication since they leave a film of oil on the skin. Or you may be happier with cleansing creams or lotions. Some of our models use a cleanser or makeup remover and *then* wash with soap. You'll have to decide for yourself the routine that's best for you. Vibeke, for example, who doesn't believe in "fancy" cosmetics and skin-care products, removes her makeup with cold cream, smearing it on with her fingers. She wipes it off with damp cotton and then washes with mild soap and water.

> **EVA VOORHIS** *swears almond oil is great for removing makeup. For Maggie Fahy, the girl with the super-sensitive skin, it's moisturizer because makeup removers make her skin break out. Cheri La Rocque, whose skin is exceptionally dry, is an advocate of petroleum jelly. "Cheap and effective," she says. So is vegetable shortening.*

Shari Belafonte, who sings like her father and models Calvin Klein jeans on TV, also uses petroleum jelly to remove makeup, then wipes that off with alcohol on a cotton pad. "I live by Vaseline," she says.

THE FORD MODELS' SIX-STEP SKIN PROGRAM

The following is the daily routine that we recommend to our models with normal (not too dry, not too oily) skin. We'll get to specific problems later.

**STEP
1**

**STEP
2**

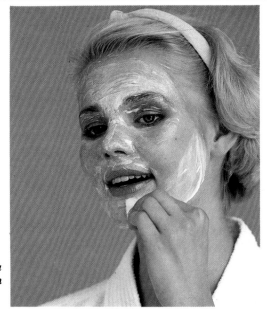

*Anna
Magnusson*

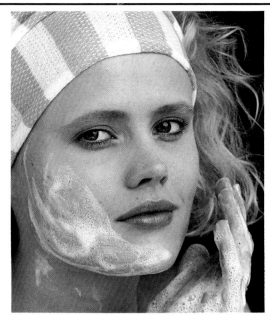

*Eva
Johansson*

CLEANSING

With some kind of makeup remover or cleanser, remove every trace of makeup from your face. Massage the cleanser in gently. Remove with damp cotton.

WASHING

Wash gently with warm water and a very mild soap. I like castile which I buy in huge blocks and cut up into cakes, but many dermatologists recommend plain, pure soap for oily or normal skin and the superfatted kinds for dryer skin. There are also no-soap soaps that are essentially detergents and tend to be less drying and/or irritating. Never use deodorant soap on your face unless your doctor has prescribed it. It's too harsh. If you have extremely dry skin, skip the soap and use only cleansing cream, then wash gently with your fingertips or a soft washcloth. If you have very oily skin, wash with soap two or three times a day, rinsing carefully.

STEP 3

STEP 4

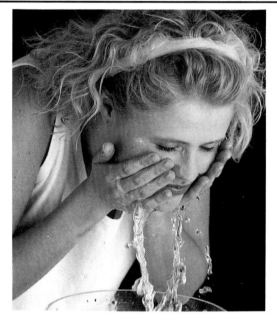

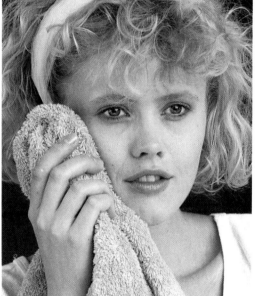

(BOTH)
Eva Johansson

RINSING

Rinse with cool or warm water at least 20 times, cupping the water in your hands. Hot water is drying.

DRYING

Pat dry with a terry towel. Don't rub.

BUTTERMILK TONER: *To tone and moisturize, try dabbing on butter-milk (wash it off in five minutes). Several of our models think it's as good as anything else for skin freshening, though Donna Stia tones with rose water.*

STEP
5

STEP
6

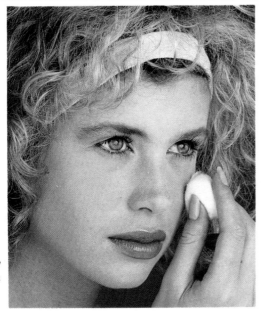

*Hayley
Mortison*

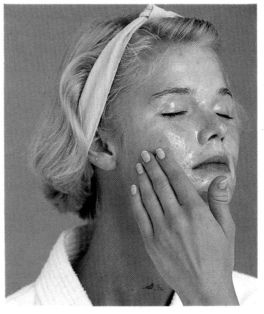

*Anna
Magnusson*

FRESHENING

Apply a mild skin freshener or toner (sometimes called a refining lotion). Try chilling it in the refrigerator. It cleanses off the last traces of makeup and soap and makes your skin feel good. Unless you're very oily, it's a good idea to dilute it to about half-strength. If you run out of freshener, substitute diluted apple-cider vinegar. It works, according to Glynnis Jones. Witch hazel is excellent, too. Rinse with cool water.

Never use harsh, excessively drying products, even if your skin is exceedingly oily. They will stimulate your oil glands to work even harder.

MOISTURIZING

Always apply moisturizer on a skin that's had a chance to absorb some water in the preceding minute. If you've just washed, leave your face slightly damp. (Anette Stai holds a washcloth under hot water, wrings it out, holds it on her face for about 30 seconds, then splashes with cold water before putting on her moisturizer in a few light coats, letting it dry in between.)

Apply the moisturizer all over your face and neck if your skin is dry or normal, at least three times a day if it's super dry, using an oil-based product. Use a water-based moisturizer only on the dry areas if your skin is oily.

You can use the same moisturizer day and night, though some models prefer a heavier, creamier night cream at bedtime.

Now you are ready for makeup (unless you're going to bed).

STEP
7

FOR DRY SKIN ONLY: LUBRICATING

Dry skin requires greasing up after washing
(unless you're applying makeup next) and
especially before going to bed. Peanut oil,
mineral oil and lanolin work fine. So do
many other products. Christie Brinkley is a
petroleum-jelly fan. At night she always
smears it on her mouth and anywhere else
that feels dry. Juli Foster uses vitamin E oil
once a week at bedtime to keep her skin soft
and supple, and Cheri La Rocque finds aloe
vera jelly does the job. She keeps it in the
refrigerator, uses it every day under her
moisturizer.

Susan Smith's father is a dermatologist
who says vegetable shortening is fine if you
run out of fancier night-time emollients. Just
rub it on gently and then wipe off the excess
with a tissue. Susan carries a stick of lip
balm in her bag for daytime use, smears it
anywhere on her face that may feel dry.
Other models use cocoa butter the same
way.

Or, if you like, you can buy marvelous
skin-care lubricants that may cost more
money but may make you feel more beautiful.

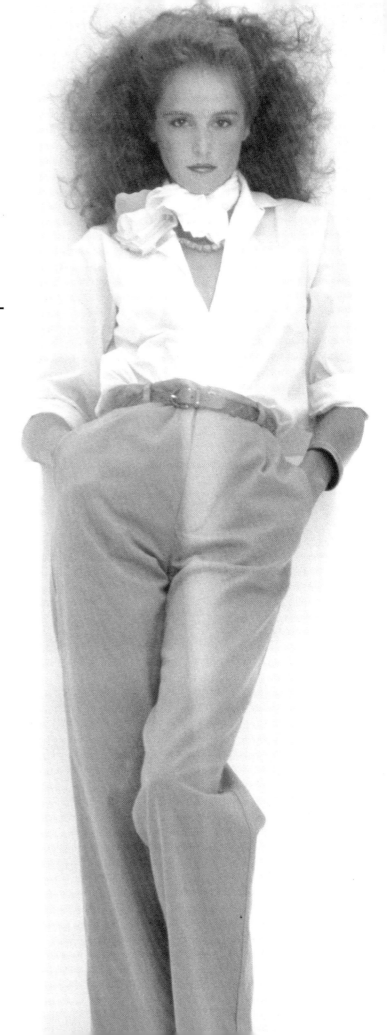

Alda

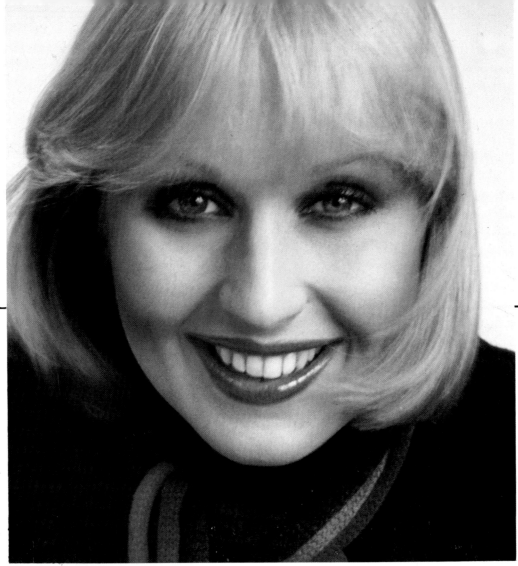

Chris Royer

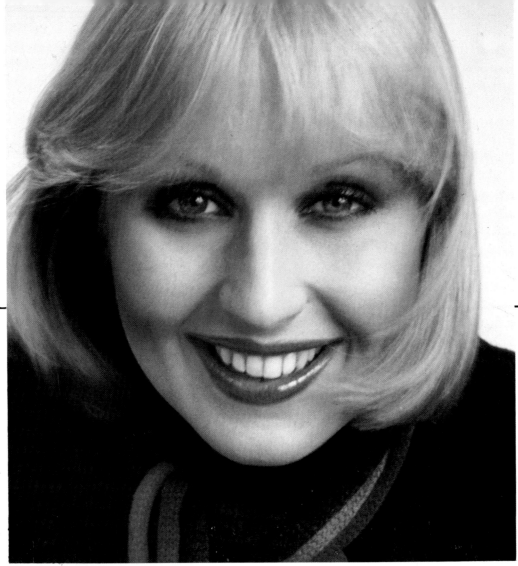 **SAUNA SOAK:** *Nancy DeWeir keeps her skin soft with this routine. She slathers plenty of moisturizer all over her face and entire body and then goes into the sauna for 10 minutes to help it soak in.*

Nancy's first booking while she was still in high school was for the cover of Seventeen, *but her career almost foundered right at the start because the shooting was scheduled for the day of her senior prom and she refused to go to the photographer's studio. I couldn't believe it, because to me, nothing is more important than a big booking. Fortunately, a compassionate editor changed the date of the shooting and Nancy did the cover. That was the start of her spectacular career.*

JACKI ADAMS, *the Florida high-school girl who now has an exclusive contract with Elizabeth Arden, likes to use different moisturizers in different seasons and always a heavier cream around her eyes. In winter, she picks an oil-based product for protection against dehydration. In summer, she prefers water-based because it's cooler.*

ALDA BALESTRA'S ROUTINE: *Our Italian beauty, Alda, lubricates her skin with night cream—but only for half an hour. Then she wipes it off to give her skin a chance to "breathe." This is good advice for anyone with extremely sensitive skin like hers.*

STEAMING YOUR FACE

Give your face a steam bath. It softens and relaxes your pores and gives them a good cleaning. Besides, it loosens up debris, including the clogged oil plugs that can become blackheads. Even better, steaming is another way to hydrate your skin. Once a week will do for normal skin; two or three times a week really helps oily or blemished skin.

Here's how: Heat water in an open pot, then let it cool a little. Place the pot on a firm surface, away from the edge, handle turned away from you. Drape a towel over your head and lean over the steam rising from the hot water. Not too close! Stay over the pot for five minutes, coming up for air now and then.

Plain steaming water is fine, but try adding some aromatic herbs or a little camomile tea. That's even better.

IF DONNA STIA *is scheduled for a beauty shot the next morning, she steams her face, adding four tablespoons of rosemary to the pot.*

If you can afford it, buy a facial sauna. Or just sit in front of the sink, turn on the hot water, drape a towel over your head and the basin and let the vapor steam your face.

LAURA ROBERSON, *who has exquisite skin, not only steams her face, she steams her entire self once a week. Laura goes to a steam bath, sits in it for about 20 minutes while drinking lots of water. This way she hydrates her whole body and "clears out impurities" at the same time.*

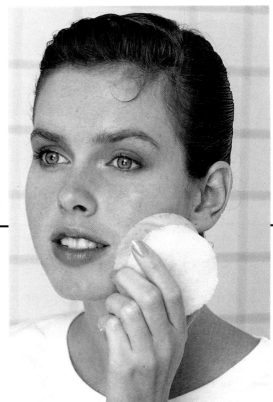

Kathy Law

POLISHING YOUR SKIN

I believe in "polishing" your skin. It rubs away the top layer of dull dead cells, along with dirt and remnants of makeup, leaving a glowing face and body that reflect more light from a smoother, moister surface.

Skin polishing should be done once or twice a week, no more, and gently at that. I don't believe in granular scrubs, even if some of our models do, but prefer using a facial sponge or puff to carefully scrub away dead cells. And I like to use it with soap or just plain warm water, though some models chose cleansing cream.

Caution: Don't be too vigorous. Never rub pimples, and don't go near your eyes. Don't do this at all if you end up with red and splotchy skin that feels battered no matter how gentle you are. You're the delicate type, and this is all too much for you!

Willow Bay, the girl in the Estée Lauder ads, polishes her skin with a scrub once a week. She likes a grainy product. Christie Brinkley has a concoction she recommends when you run out of your purchased supply and are feeling desperate: Mix a little granulated sugar with soap and apply with *cool* water (so the sugar doesn't dissolve). Cristina Ferrare doesn't believe in harsh facial treatments. A couple of times a week, she gives her face a very mild honey-and-almond scrub. You can make your own by mixing ground almonds with a little honey and perhaps adding a touch of moisturizer. Donna Stia uses a natural sea sponge as an exfoliator. Erin Gray, the star of a TV series, likes an apricot scrub and a soft sponge.

Chemical exfoliants are the newest kind of skin polishers and are usually mild enough to use every day. You spread them on your skin where they dissolve the dead surface cells, before washing them off.

COPING WITH BLEMISHES

Everybody gets blemishes—even models. Most models have professional facials about once a month. The steaming and the special masks and the blackhead treatments are very helpful. In between, they give themselves facials.

Every one of our girls has her own routine for coverup and cure. But before we get to their personal discoveries, here's what I recommend. My advice is based on information I have gathered from many prominent dermatologists. I am talking about normal skin here—if you have problem skin, see our section on acne.

To get rid of blackheads: Steam your face. Then gently, gently, gently squeeze the loosened blackhead with two fingers buffered with tissue. Never squeeze hard. Never force it. Never pinch. If it doesn't yield to your fingers readily, forget it. Rinse 30 times with cool water. Now, if you have the time, apply a mask—a beaten egg will do—to close the pores and soothe the skin.

ANETTE STAI, *who comes from Norway, is full of advice for looking good. One of her tips is the fast blackhead eradicator: "Instead of steaming my face, I wet a washcloth with really hot water and press it on the area, rewetting as needed, until the skin is softened and the pores relax. Then the blackhead usually pops right out. I finish up with a really cold washcloth that helps eliminate the redness."*

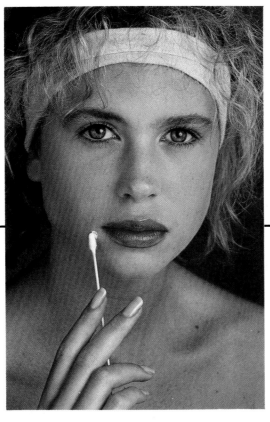

Hayley Mortison

Don't fool around with whiteheads or real pimples, or you may make them a lot worse. Never try to squeeze them. You can, however, try to get pimples to open up and heal more quickly by applying hot compresses, then dabbing them with a drying lotion. There are many excellent medicated products for this purpose. Homemade drying agents include alcohol or lemon juice (mix with water and dot on the spot once a day).

> **TO SOOTHE AND SMOOTH,**
> *Nancy DeWeir buys aloe vera juice in a health-food store and uses it as a skin lotion to keep her skin clear.*

SENSIBLE SKIN STRATEGIES

If you get many blemishes constantly, blame overactive and irritated oil glands, triggered by who knows what. The causes usually named are excess hormones, tension, heredity, the menstrual cycle, birth-control pills, insufficient rest, certain kinds of cosmetics, and foods. Some women consistently break out if they use a rich moisturizer or night cream or use it too often. The heavy oil clogs their pores. Facials do it for Nancy DeWeir. Cleansing cream does it for other people. Try products that are water-based and use them only on dry areas. Perfumed products make Renée Simonsen break out so she always sniffs before she buys. They are also drying. Carrie Miller, Renee Russo, and Eva Voorhis share the same problem. Kim Charlton has discovered that old makeup makes her skin erupt so she thows it out after a couple of months.

Always keep your skin scrupulously clean, especially after a workout when your sweat and oil glands work overtime, and check your diet to be sure it is balanced and healthy and includes plenty of fruits and vegetables.

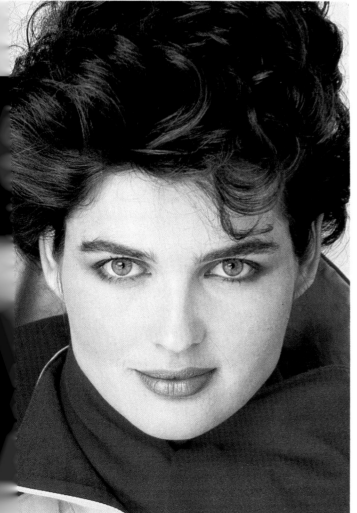

BANNING BLEMISHES: *So she doesn't dry out areas of her face that don't need it, Christie Brinkley dots a little oily-skin mask on her minor blemishes, lets it dry, then rinses it off. She says it works.*

EMERGENCY REMEDY *from Ty Hendrick: If you see signs of breaking out, start drinking lots of water with lemon juice to flush out your system. Ty also takes a small dose (30 mg) of zinc supplement occasionally at bedtime in an effort to ward off outbreaks.*

Eva Voorhis

COVERING UP

There are so many coverup products available today that you can always find one that works for you. Most models use an under-makeup drying lotion twice a day to speed healing, then cover up with skin-toned medication or a coverup stick before applying a sheer foundation.

"It's not that models don't break out," says Vibeke. "Sure they do. The only difference is they learn how to cover up. For work, what I do is make a pimple into a beauty spot. First I put on a drying lotion, then I cover it with brown pencil just like a little beauty mark."

RAMPANT AMONG MODELS *is a trick I'd never heard of—a dab of toothpaste to dry up a blemish. Nancy DeWeir says it clears hers up quicker than anything. "The next morning it's usually gone. It's not your run-of-the-mill beauty treatment, but it sure works in a pinch." Patricia Van Ryckeghem, on the other hand, prefers alcohol, then covers over with a little makeup. Patricia, by the way, comes from Belgium. Her doting grandmother entered her in a beauty contest which she won and that was the start of her modeling career.*

SPECIAL FOR SERIOUS ACNE

If your skin is truly bad, you require the services of a dermatologist. Ask about vitamin A acid cream, benzoyl peroxide, and topical antibiotics. Occasionally, antibiotics taken internally are prescribed. Be especially careful to be in optimum health. Eat a low-fat, low-sugar, balanced, nutritious diet.

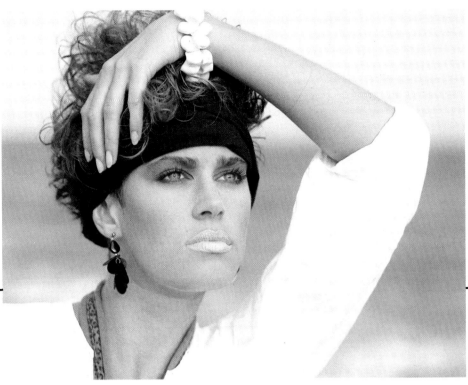

Carrie Miller

- Wash your face twice a day with a special medicated soap. Some doctors recommend deodorant soap because of its antibacterial action, but ask yours before you try it. Avoid the scented varieties which may be irritating to your already irritated skin. Do not use cleansing cream.

- Rinse well and follow with a toner to be sure you get all residue off.

- Clean your skin immediately after a workout. Carry some astringent towelettes with you, then wash when you get home.

- Don't do any do-it-yourself squeezing, pressing, poking, or picking. Hands off. If any of this should be done, let the dermatologist attend to it.

- Avoid anything that may be irritating, such as steaming and facial scrubbing or exfoliating.

- Try gently rubbing some ice over your face. This may help reduce any swelling and inflammation around the more serious blemishes.

- Choose water-based skin-care products and cosmetics. Use powder blush rather than cream.

- Avoid heavy sources of iodine (or iodide), such as iodized salt.

FACE-SAVING MASKS

I recommend that our models use a mask once a week, choosing one designed for their skin type. Masks remove dull, lusterless surface cells, deep-clean the pores, remove traces of makeup and dirt. Some masks temporarily plump up your skin, others rev up circulation or tighten. Whatever kind you use, you're sure to have smoother, softer, more alive skin.

Masks for dry skin are rich and creamy and full of moisturizing ingredients. They remove dead cells but don't strip away moisture and oil. Oily-skin masks are usually made of drying agents like clay or mud that deep-clean and remove excess oil.

AN ADVOCATE OF YOGURT MASKS *is Evelyn Kuhn, a model I discovered on one of my scouting trips to Germany. Evelyn pats yogurt all over her face and neck, leaves it on for half an hour, rinses it off, and swears it makes her dry skin clean and smooth. In winter when her skin gets really dry, she alternates the yogurt routine with a mixture of honey and egg yolks which she says hydrates her skin.*

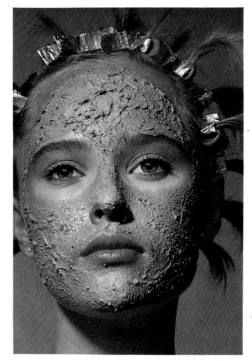

Kerstin Marie

Always read the directions that come with the mask you buy because they differ. But here is the usual procedure:

**STEP
1**

Cleanse your face thoroughly.

**STEP
2**

Give your face a steaming.

**STEP
3**

Apply eye cream around your eyes to protect that delicate area.

**STEP
4**

If your skin is extremely dry, apply a light coating of moisturizer all over your face and neck.

**STEP
5**

With upward and outward feathery strokes, spread the mask lightly all over your face, except around your eyes and lips. Lie down, preferably with your feet high and your head low to increase circulation to your face. Place cotton pads soaked in camomile tea (or thin slices of cucumber) on your eyes, and think pleasant thoughts for 15 minutes (or for however long the directions prescribe).

**STEP
6**

Wet a washcloth with warm water and press it to your face to soften the hardened mask. Rinse with warm water. Pat dry. Apply moisturizer on damp skin.

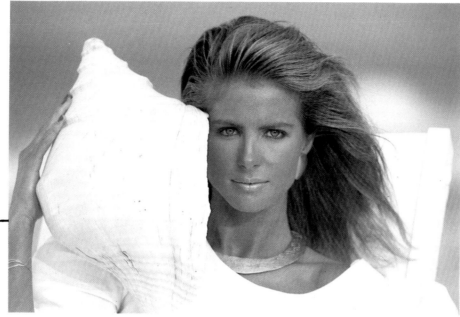

Cheri La Rocque

KITCHEN CONCOCTIONS

Here are concoctions to put together at home if you don't want to spend the money on a commercial mask or if you've run out of it. We've collected the recipes from Ford models.

For dry skin:

- Egg yolk, one teaspoon of almond oil, one tablespoon of honey.

- Egg yolk, plain. Let it dry for 20 minutes.

- Mashed avocado spread over your face for half an hour. That's Cheri La Rocque's favorite.

- Egg yolk mixed with two teaspoons of vegetable oil.

- Cucumber juice. Nina Renshaw cuts a cucumber into very thin slices, twists them in a big handkerchief, squeezing out the juice into a bowl and storing it in the refrigerator to use as a mask. Other models just place cucumber slices on their faces.

CHRIS ROYER, *who models for all the top fashion houses, likes to travel light. For a quick mask, she orders up some yogurt and honey from room service, mixes together a teaspoon of each, and smooths it over her face. It's especially effective, she says, in hot, humid climates.*

For oily skin:

- Two egg whites mixed with a few drops of lemon juice. Or just plain egg whites.

- Brewer's yeast with a few drops of water to make a paste.

- Rolled oats, oatmeal or almond meal mixed with enough warm water to form a paste.

- Two tablespoons honey, one teaspoon lemon juice in a tablespoon of hot water.

DEBRA HALLEY'S TINGLY TREAT-MENT *is Vicks VapoRub, something the rest of us may use for chest colds. Debra, discovered while waiting on tables in a tiny Western town, says, "I wash my face with mild soap, pat it almost dry, then use VapoRub down the middle of my face where it's oiliest. I've found it keeps my skin tight and shiny and fresh."*

FORD SOLUTIONS FOR SPECIAL SKIN PROBLEMS:

PUFFY EYES: If you wake up in the morning, and you've got a pair of puffy eyes, try applying ice cubes wrapped in a wet washcloth. That works for me. Glynnis Jones makes a strong camomile tea, chills it, lies down with soaked cotton balls on her eyes. Nina Renshaw recommends tea bags soaked in boiling water, then put into the freezer for 15 minutes. The cheaper the tea, the better, because of its higher level of tannic acid.

UNDER-EYE PUFFS: Don't use heavy creams or oily substances around your eyes before you go to bed. Instead, use a lighter cream during the day. If you're a big salt consumer, cut back. Your bags may be due to fluid retention. See makeup chapter for camouflage.

CHAPPED LIPS: Chapped lips are truly avoidable. All you have to do is keep lipstick or lip balm or gloss on them—or lip sunscreen in the sun. There are also those special lip primers that prevent chapping as well as runny lipstick.

If, like the rest of us, you sometimes get chapped lips despite all precautions, try this trick offered by Maggie Fahy. It's one she learned from a makeup artist when she arrived on location with rough lips. Take a toothbrush, soften it in hot water, and brush your lips gently. Pat on light moisturizer, oil or cream. Wipe gently.

When your lips are chapped, don't use bright or deep lipsticks. Use clear glossy lip products, and play up the rest of your face.

> **THE GIRL STRETCHED OUT** on all those Coppertone billboards is Donna Sexton, who's famous for her body as well as her face. "I'm a firm believer in lip balm," Donna states. "I keep it by my bed, by the phone, everywhere."

ROUGH ELBOWS: You may not see your elbows, but everybody else does, so pay attention to them. To get rid of rough skin, fill a little bowl with warm water and a teaspoon of dishwashing detergent. Soak each elbow in it for about ten minutes. Now use a facial scrub to remove the rough skin. Rinse. Use body lotion or a polishing pad.

To eliminate dark skin, cut a lemon in two and stick an elbow in each half for 20 minutes or so. Rinse. Apply body lotion.

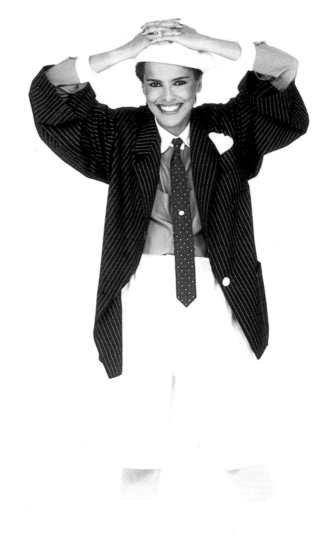

Shari Belafonte

BROWN SPOTS: Always use a sunscreen to prevent more of them. Try an over-the-counter bleaching cream or a stronger one your dermatologist can prescribe. Check with the doctor about removing brown spots with dermabrasion, electrodessication (burning with an electric needle), or cryotherapy (freezing).

DILATED CAPILLARIES: Try electrodessication applied by a dermatologist. It hardly hurts, and it usually works. Peeling agents, again applied by a physician, are another method of attack as are "sclerosing" injections. Facial masks that contain vasoconstrictors make capillaries less noticeable. Meantime, you can cover them up with coverup cream and/or foundation. A slight green tinge to the base will help disguise the redness. Don't use abrasive facial scrubs.

VERY SENSITIVE SKIN: Avoid products containing perfumes or alcohol. Carrie Peterson, who gets rashes if she's not careful, also stays away from very oily products and iridescent eye makeup, which she doesn't like anyway. Nancy DeWeir's skin can't take facials or scrubs or most masks. Watch out for heavy creams and cleansing lotions.

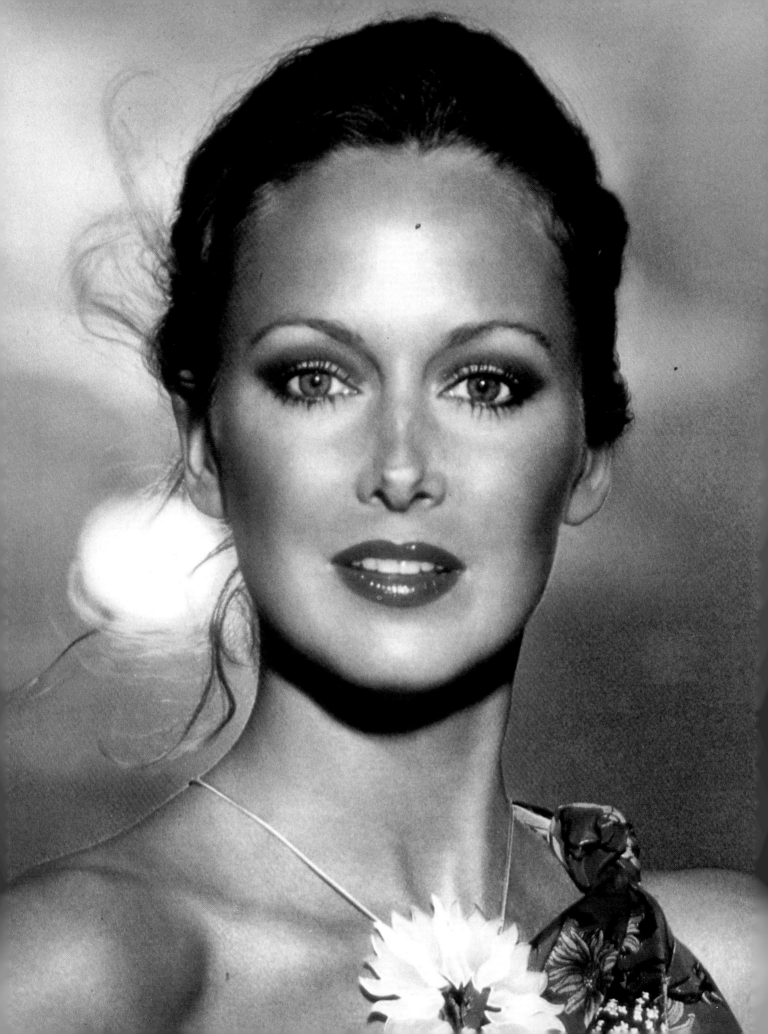

HOW TO REDESIGN YOUR FACE WITH MAKEUP

There's *nobody* who doesn't look better with makeup, including the best models. Professional models probably know more about the art of makeup than anyone else in the world, because they practice their art daily. For most photographic shootings and fashion shows, they apply their own cosmetics. If a girl has many bookings in a day, she may have to change her look two or three times, and she must be pretty quick because time is money in our business. Models get paid by the hour, and clients don't like to be kept waiting.

Our new models attend classes at the agency so they can start out fast. No girl can go on a booking without knowing the basics, because there's often no money in the client's budget for a makeup artist. Our reputation depends on our models' professionalism. On most jobs, they are asked to come with "hair and makeup ready." That is noted on their charts by our bookers and passed along to the models when they call in the late afternoon for the following day's assignments. "Makeup" usually means basic makeup that may be altered at the studio, depending on the shot and the needs of the client. For instance, at one sitting a girl may need makeup for evening, at the next she may be wearing a swimsuit.

When girls start going out on bookings, they learn even more from makeup artists who are hired on high-budget jobs to redesign their faces for the camera. The new models quickly discover that makeup *is* magic. Skillfully applied, it can literally create the impression of perfection for you too. It can give you wonderful coloring, better proportions, flawless skin. It plays up your best features and deemphasizes your flaws. It creates illusion.

LOOKING GOOD, LOOKING NATURAL

Good makeup today is light-textured and natural. It doesn't look like it's been painted on, and it isn't plastered over your face like a mask. It simply

Karen Graham

makes you look great. That means you may be wearing a lot of makeup, but it doesn't show. Designer Ralph Lauren says, "I never like to see makeup during the day. I just want to see beautiful coloring, good bones. The idea is to be light-handed, to look good out-of-doors without looking made up." I agree. Always underplay except for extravagant nighttime occasions.

Lacey Ford puts it this way: "When you look at yourself in a mirror, you don't see makeup. You see your eyes look bigger, your cheeks look a little rosier. You have a healthy glow, your skin looks clear, and you have wonderful bones. It's all got to be very subtle. At night, for special occasions, you can use cosmetics as an interesting accessory, but even then, you should look purposely exaggerated only for a special effect."

What's more, the older you are, the less makeup you should wear. Overdone cosmetics *add* years rather than take them away. Erin Gray, who is in her thirties and is now a television celebrity, says she's been wearing less and less, applying only what's needed to "correct" her features—like enlarging her eyes and softening her natural cupid's-bow mouth—except on special occasions.

Speaking of special occasions, Patricia Van Ryckeghem wears very little makeup most of the time but changes radically when she goes out dancing. One of her favorite combinations is blue lips and green blusher! My advice: If you like way-out makeup, be sure you enjoy causing a sensation. Most of these trendy tricks are only for the very young.

THE MODEL'S LIFE

Models never go out in the evening with the same makeup they've worn all day. When they come home from work, the first thing they do is remove it. If they're going out again, they will recreate their faces with a great deal less makeup than they needed for photography.

Everybody thinks models go around exquisitely made up. They don't. In fact, most of them wear no makeup, or hardly any, when they are not working. Renée Simonsen, among the most beautiful girls I've ever seen, says she keeps her face completely clean for real life except for mascara. Kathryn Redding wears a little makeup, because, she says, her face needs definition. "My coloring is so pale," Kathryn says, "that I always wear a trace of

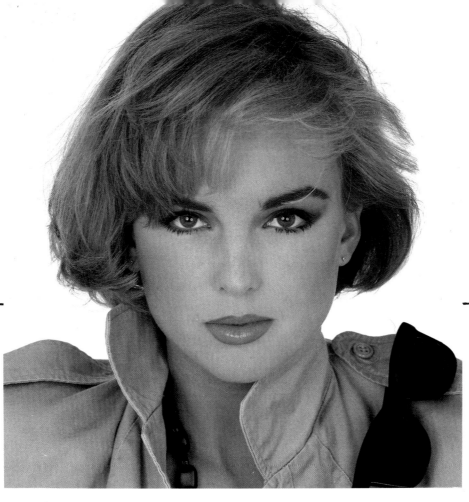

Julie Floyd

blusher and some mascara, plus eyebrow pencil." Kim Charlton is another who wears eye makeup, just a little, because she's so fair. Blond and wide-eyed, Kim is married to our executive vice president, Joe Hunter, who heads our Ford Men division.

Vibeke's another who says, "No work, no makeup, unless I'm going some-where. Then I use less makeup, less intense, more subtle, well blended. I don't exaggerate it as I do for photography. I like to look natural." Jacki Adams, the girl who appears in all the Elizabeth Arden ads and commer-cials, likes her skin to breathe and wears only the lightest foundation when she's off the job. Vanessa Angel, the tall, lanky British beauty discovered in a London restaurant, also rests her face between bookings. "I spend all day made up," Vanessa explains. "When I'm not working, forget it."

THE NO-MAKEUP LOOK *is what Martha Longley strives for, too. "I only use a little foundation in the winter when my skin has no color from the sun, plus some blusher and mascara. That's it!"*

Take a tip from these working models and go around makeup-free when you can. It gives your skin a breather. When you do apply makeup, remem-ber to make it look subtle. Keep it natural. Save the obvious for big nights on the town.

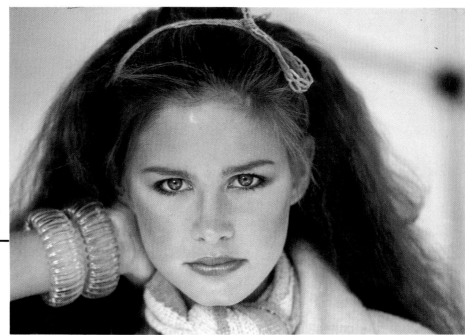

Juli Foster

NO MAJOR MYSTERY

Applying makeup artfully may seem a major mystery, but it's really quite simple when you use the techniques we teach our models. Once you understand what to do, then you must practice, practice, practice. Learn one technique before going on to another. Do it over and over again until your hand is sure and steady. It usually takes one of our new models about two weeks to master the magic of makeup. That's with intense motivation, because the success of her new career depends on it. It may take you a little longer, but you will learn.

Don't buy any cosmetics untried, unless you enjoy throwing money away. Go to a beauty counter, put on the makeup, and see how you like it. If you don't find what you want, walk away and try other products at other counters. Don't feel you must buy until you are sure. Makeup is expensive, and the only way to choose is by experimenting.

NEEDED: AN HONEST APPRAISAL

To apply makeup artfully, you must know what your face really looks like. Study your face from all angles and in all kinds of light, until you know quite objectively what your good and bad features are.

Christie Brinkley says, "I always put my daytime makeup on sitting in natural light, near a window." I suggest you do the same, since that's the light in which you'll probably be seen when you leave the house. Check your finished job by the window with a big mirror. It's all too easy to step out into the bright sunlight looking ready for the chorus line.

If you must use artificial light, pure white incandescent bulbs are the best if they are bright enough for you to see exactly what you are doing. Fluorescent lights are the worst. They make you look washed out and slightly green, and you'll tend to compensate by overdoing your makeup.

THE FORD MODELS' MAKEUP PLAN

Here is the way we advise our models to apply their makeup—the details come later. You will see the gradual transformation of Renée Simonsen as a top makeup artist demonstrates the proper techniques for a natural daytime look. Put yourself in Renée's place.

STEP 1	**STEP 2**

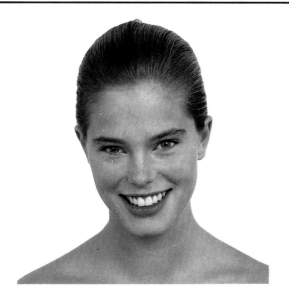 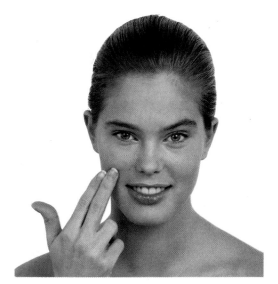

Here you are without makeup, cleansed and scrubbed, with only a coat of moisturizer between you and the world.

Apply coverup cream to the circles under your eyes, to dark areas near your nose or at the sides of your mouth, and over any red or blotchy areas. Remember to cover the hollows between your nose and your inner eye corner. It's best to use a coverup that's the same as your own skin tone or just a half-shade lighter. If it is too light, it will look obvious or gray; too dark, you'll look unreal.

Model for pages 49–53: Renée Simonsen

Makeup by Kevyn Aucoin.

STEP 3

STEP 4

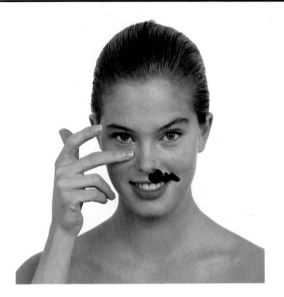

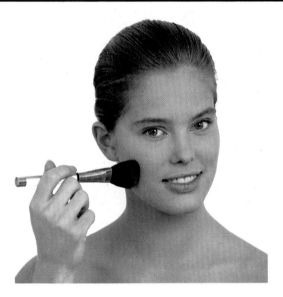

Apply a *light* film of foundation (base) all over your face (including those areas where you've used coverup), blending it carefully. Use a water-based liquid foundation for oily or normal skin, and oil-based for dry skin. Dot it all over your face with your fingertips. Then, using your fingers or a slightly damp sponge (dampened with water for water-based, moisturizer for oil-based), blend it outwards and upwards, all the way into the hairline and down just under the chin line. Don't extend foundation all over the neck because it never looks natural and it gets on your clothes. If you've chosen the right shade, one that truly matches your own skin color, you won't need it anyway.

NOTE: Foundations look darker in the bottle than they do on you. Match your base to the skin on your cheek just above your jawline, not your hand or your wrist which is a different color. Remember, you'll need a different foundation when you have a tan.

With a brush or a cotton ball, dust translucent powder all over your face to produce a matte finish and set the foundation. *Important.*

STEP 5

STEP 6

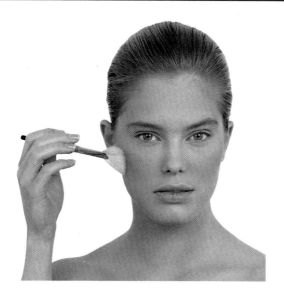

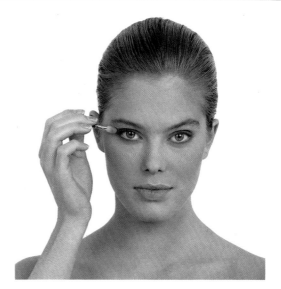

Now apply blusher as explained on pp. 62–67. The big tendency is to use too much. You should look as if you have your own natural rosy cheeks. Add a little at the temples.

Smudge matte powder eyeshadow (this makeup artist prefers brown) under your eyes near the lashes. Use a sponge application, tapping it or blowing on it first to get rid of the excess. Now blend it over your eyelids right up to your brows, darker near your eye and diminishing in intensity to almost nothing at the browbones. Line your eyes with a dark pencil as close to your lashes as possible and smudge it with a sponge applicator or a finger to create a smoky effect. *Important.*

STEP 7

STEP 8

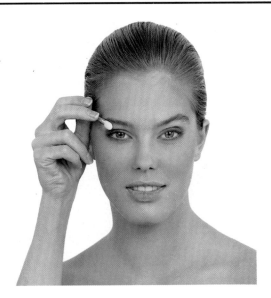

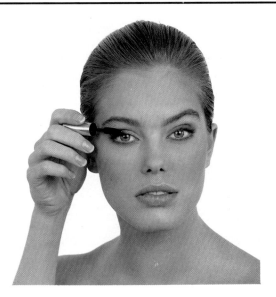

Apply highlighter (matte beige) just under the browbone. A touch will do. It's also nice just on the top of your cheekbone.

Apply black mascara to top and bottom lashes.

STEP 9

STEP 10

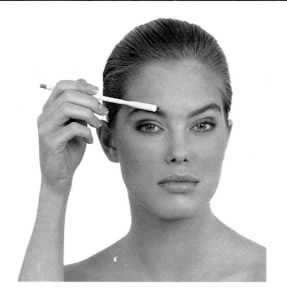

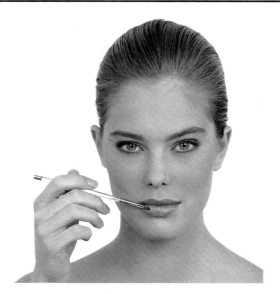

Fill in your eyebrows, if necessary, using a pencil that matches or is slightly lighter than your natural color. Brush them out so they don't look too heavy.

If your lipstick tends to run, smooth on some lip primer and let it dry. Shape your lips with a lip pencil. Then fill in the rest of your mouth with the same pencil. With a lipbrush, apply lipstick over the pencil. Blot lips with a tissue to matte the color and increase its staying power. Apply gloss if you like.

FORD MODELS' MAKEUP SECRETS

All Ford models have learned how to make impressive improvements on what God gave them. Follow their advice and see what makeup can do for you.

COVERUP: Coverup cream is one of the handiest cosmetics ever invented. Pat it on very gently and blend it just enough to conceal whatever it is you want to hide. Eveyn Kuhn uses it every day for dark circles under her eyes. You can use it on dark pigment, little red blemishes, recessed areas that cast shadows where you don't want them. The secret is a light touch.

Makeup artist Timothy Metz suggests applying concealer with a small artist's brush. "You can paint out dark areas or blemishes with much more control than using your fingers," he says. "Dip the brush into the concealer, wipe most of it off and then paint."

> **CLOTILDE, THE RALPH LAUREN** *girl from Norway who is now making movies, chooses an ivory tone of foundation as a coverup for her dark circles, and then blends her regular shade over it.*

SKINTONE CORRECTORS: If your skin is too sallow, too ruddy, too colorless, too anything, and you don't like it, use a color wash (underbase, primer, subtint) to correct it before putting on your foundation. It works wonders. It looks natural. Many of our models wear a wash without any foundation over it when they're not working because it gives a nice healthy glow and nobody will ever know you're wearing anything.

For sallow greenish or yellowish skin, use a light film of lavender or mauve underbase. Try peach or apricot if you're extremely pallid and color-less. I like green corrector for ruddy complexions that have too much red-ness. Pure white neutralizes any tone. You can use corrector only where you need it if your skin tends to have reddish blotches or dilated capillaries you'd like to camouflage. Always apply it sparingly, blending it well.

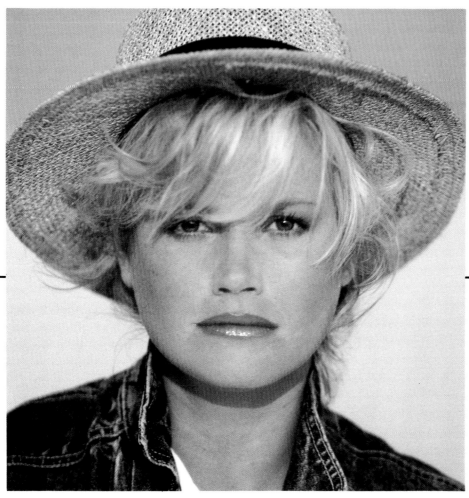

Maggie Fahy

FOUNDATION: Even if your skin is perfect, you need foundation. It should match your skin tone. If it doesn't, you won't look real. And it must be muted. It can have a *slightly* rosy tone if you're sallow, or it can be *slightly* beige or green if you're ruddy. But only slightly. If you alter the tone more than that, you'll look painted. The purpose of base is to make your skin look flawless, not to change its color. Vibeke, for example, uses very little foundation on her face but chooses a color just half a shade *paler* than her own skin because, she says, it gives a younger, more perfect finish.

Always apply your foundation lightly and sheerly, blending it carefully right into your hairline and down just under your chin so there's not a line or a streak or a vacancy anywhere.

Most of our models use liquid foundation. It is sheerer and more transparent than cream. You can make it even sheerer by adding moisturizer to oil-based and water to water-based foundation. Pour some of the liquid into your palm and add just a drop or two of the thinner until it's the right texture. Put it on with your fingertips or a damp sponge. Anette Stai mixes water with her lotion and smooths it over her face with a sponge, stopping right under her chinline, for a sheer matte finish.

For smooth coverage, always let your moisturizer set for about five minutes before applying foundation. Never apply the base in a thick, heavy coat, even when you're trying to conceal shadows or flaws. For extra coverage, use additional thin coats, letting them dry in between, building up very subtly in the areas where you need it.

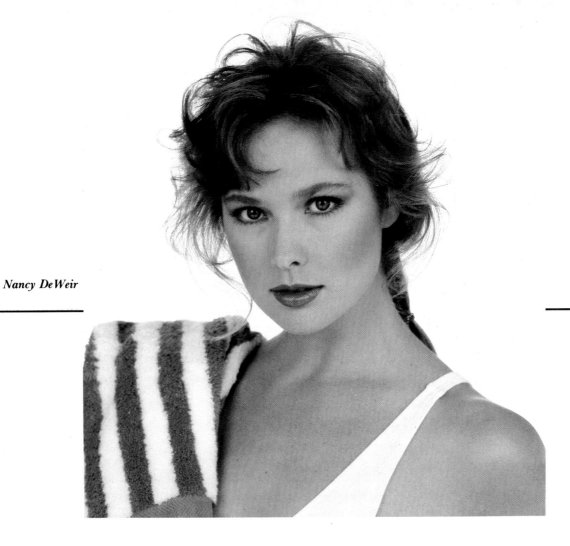

Nancy DeWeir

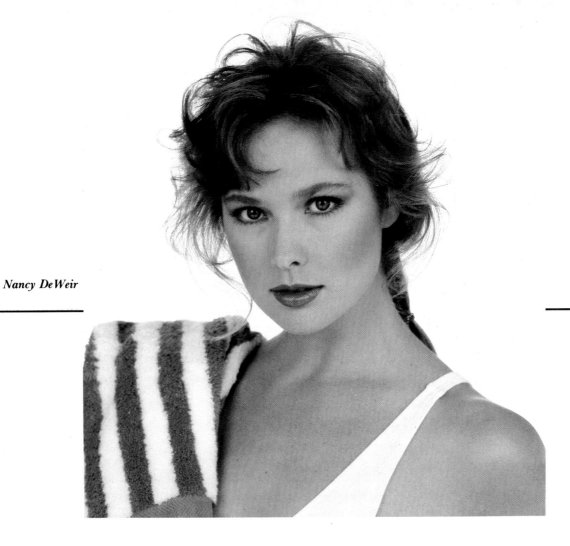

ARE YOU A FRECKLE FACE?

Today's look is natural, healthy, fresh, real. Freckles are part of that look, so if you've got them, enjoy them. Maggie Fahy, who has appeared in as many as 19 commercials airing at one time, says, "I have loads of freckles, and I love them. So do the clients. I never try to hide them."

   But, if your freckles are too much for you, you can block them out with a green-toned subtint under your foundation. Don't get too enthusiastic about concealing them totally, because you can't. If you feel really afflicted, see a dermatologist who can get rid of many of them for you.

OPTICAL ILLUSIONS: CONTOURING

Professional models use contouring to accent their best features and to correct flaws. Because the painted look is definitely out of fashion, it's essential to contour with extreme subtlety. That means you must practice—in natural light. It's worth the time, however, because when contouring is virtually undetectable, it can pay astonishing dividends in illusion. Caution: until you are really adept at contouring, save it for after dark.

WASH YOUR BRUSHES *once a week, says Kevyn Aucoin, makeup artist. He suggests washing with shampoo, then dipping them into hair conditioner. Leave them overnight. In the morning, rinse, towel dry, shape by hand, and air-dry, handles down.*

Donna Stia

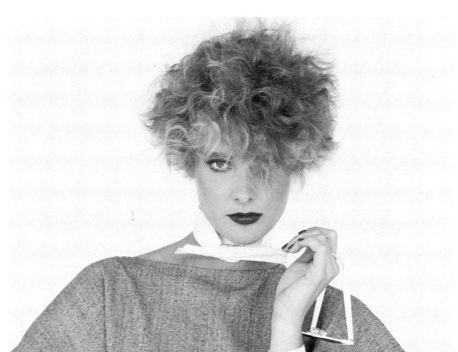

Contouring is accomplished by using a slightly darker shade of foundation, blusher, or contouring powder in the areas you want to deemphasize or hollow out, because it makes them less noticeable. And by using a slightly lighter shade on whatever you want to accent or enlarge. Apply the contour over your foundation, blend the two together extremely carefully, set with translucent powder and a spray of mineral water.

A VERY THIN FACE needs very little contouring, says Karen Bjornson, who's got one. "If I try to shape my face, I look emaciated. I use only a small amount of blusher on my cheekbones, then rub it almost off or pat powder over it."

Karen is very slender, just as all high-fashion models must be. Last season, she worked for Bill Blass, Perry Ellis, Calvin Klein, and Ralph Lauren, among others, and is now the world's highest-paid fashion-show model.

HOW THE MODELS DO IT

• **SQUARE FACE:** Vibeke claims she has a square-shaped face. To create the illusion of more roundness and less angularity, she creates shadows with pressed blusher in a brownish shade, applying it to the corners of her jaw, just under her chin, and in the corners of her wide temples. "In my personal life," Vibeke says, "I don't use much, just a little. I am very subtle, and I blend carefully so the contrast never shows. For photography, I can get much more intense and dramatic."

- **WIDE FOREHEAD:** I happen to like broad foreheads, but if you think yours is too wide or high, apply contour right along the hairline, especially at the corners. This deflects the light from this area and makes it look smaller. Cheryl Tiegs is one model who minimizes her forehead by shading along the sides and top. Very subtly, of course. Debra Halley is another. She feels her forehead looks too angular with its "bare corners." She fills the corners in with brown contouring powder the same color as her hair. Using a small stiff brush, she dabs the powder on so it looks like hair and blends with the real stuff. By the way, Debra uses more on one side than the other because that side of her forehead is higher.

- **LOW FOREHEAD:** Cover the hairline with soft hair or bangs that start far back and forget about makeup tricks. But, if you want, you can give the impression of a higher forehead by applying a *lighter* shade of foundation just along the hairline. This brings the area forward and makes it look larger.

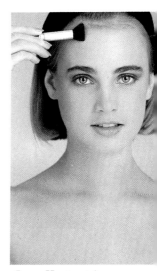

- **PROMINENT JAWLINE:** How about simply enjoying it, as Lacey Ford does? She *emphasizes* her wide jaw because she thinks it gives her face more character. She dabs lighter powder on it after applying her foundation and then blends it with a damp sponge.

If your wide or square jaw bothers you, you can do the opposite to play it down. Nancy DeWeir brushes on a faint, darker line just under the jawbone to give the impression of a more chiseled jaw. Cheryl Tiegs admits to blending brownish powder on the sides of her jaw to soften it, and also uses a little under her chin to make it look less pointed. Julie Floyd, a young model from Arizona, shades the sides of her face and her jawline for more definition.

Joyce Hartenstein

- Maggie Fahy, whom you see in so many television commercials tossing her thick, golden brown hair, uses contouring powder in a very light brown to disguise the faint signs of a double chin, dabbing it on the puffy area. "Don't try to contour your neck," she says. "Models do it for photography, but on real people it looks awful!"

- I can't think of a single Ford model with a receding chin, though there are a few who need more emphasis to make their chins appear strong.

They apply a *lighter* shade of makeup all along the jawline from ear to ear, then add a little right on the bottom of the chin.

- Do the opposite for a protruding chin. Dab a darker contour on it.

- Speaking of chins, Carrie Peterson, our only model from the Virgin Islands, has a little cleft in hers. For beauty shots she likes to accentuate it, so she takes a brush and shades it with a little fine line right down the center, then blends it almost to nothing with a fine makeup sponge. "I don't recommend contouring for the street," Carrie says, "unless you are positive it won't show."

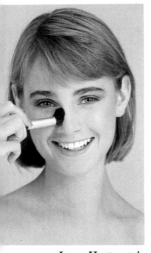

Joyce Hartenstein

- **NOW FOR NOSES:** Contouring your nose can produce dramatic optical illusions, again if you're careful not to be obvious. Use a narrow flat-edge brush, stroking on the powder and feathering the edges.

- To make your nose look slimmer, use the contour down the sides and, if needed, across the nostrils. Lighten your nose down the center.

- To make it look wider, run the shading down the center, and/or highlight the sides.

- To shorten a long nose, use just a speck of shading on the tip.

- To straighten a crooked nose, apply the shading on the crooked side and subtly highlight the straighter area.

- To soften a Roman nose, shade the most prominent part.

CHRIS ROYER, *one of Halston's favorite models, says her nose sometimes photographs too pointy. To soften it, she draws a very faint little dark line along the center of the tip, from just below the tip to just above, smudges it till it's barely there, then powders.*

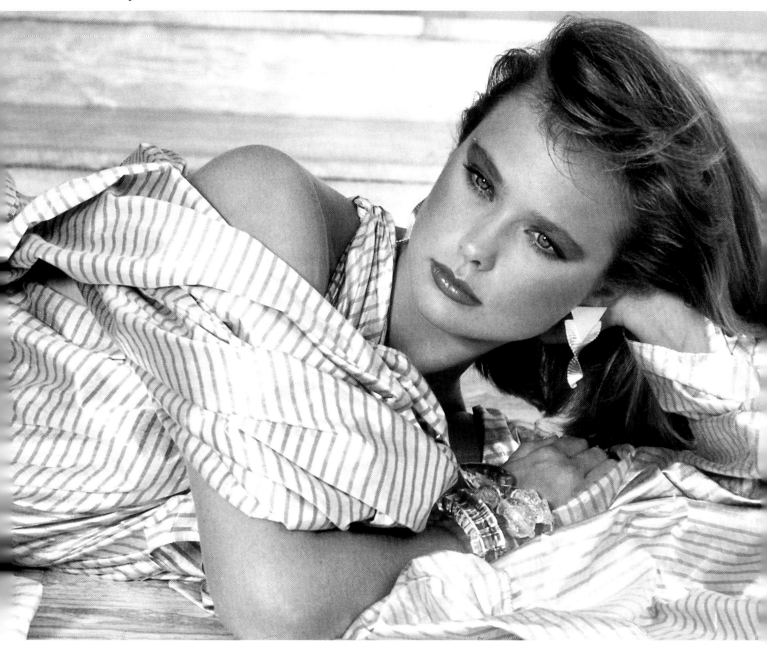

THE POWER OF POWDER

Most women don't understand the importance of powder. It gives a nice smooth matte finish to your makeup, sets it and makes it last longer, evens out tones and reduces shine. Always use loose translucent powder applied with a big soft brush or a cotton ball. Dip the brush or cotton into the powder, tap off the excess, and whisk it on. Dust off any that shows or collects in creases or corners. Models use powder whether their skin is dry or oily, but, of course, it's really essential for oily skin. Concentrate on the center of your face.

The older you are, the less powder you should use because it tends to settle in the creases. Besides, your skin becomes less oily. Confine the powder to the nose and forehead.

ALDA BALESTRA *passes along a tip she learned from a Japanese makeup artist: Apply your powder with your brush, then clap your hands near your face to remove the excess.*

I like no-color powder, but if you prefer color, be sure it's exactly the same shade as your foundation (which should be exactly the same shade as your skin). Chris Royer dusts her face with a yellowish powder "because my skin has yellow undertones, and I like it. I also use a yellowish foundation to play up my own color and to keep my neck from being different from my face. It makes me look healthy."

DEBRA HALLEY *uses baby powder to set her foundation because it's so sheer. For photography, she mixes it with face powder to reduce the sheen. "For everyday use, though, you can use it plain,"* Debra says. *"It doesn't look white if you make sure to shake off the excess from the brush first."*

THE BASICS OF BLUSHER

So many women use too much blusher, or a totally unnatural color, or both, and they look overdone. Usually the problem is the lighting where you make yourself up. In the dimness of the ordinary bathroom, you may look fantastic, but not so in the daylight. That's true of all makeup, but the major disaster areas are cheek and eye makeup.

You should look as if the makeup is really you—naturally glowing, as if you are terribly healthy, doing all the things you should do every day. For starters, choose a shade that *could* be your own. In general, the fairer your skin, the paler the blusher. Pale skin usually looks best in beigey pinks and browned corals, and sometimes a slightly rosier shade. Browner or more olive skin tends to look wonderful with bronzey, browny or peachy golden colors. Try pinching your cheeks and studying the color if you're having trouble deciding what your natural hue is.

"FOR BLUE EYES, *brown is very flattering,"* says Anette Stai who spends at least an hour every night on her beauty routines and practices different ways of putting on makeup. *"I use a brownish blusher on my eyelids, as well as on my cheeks, forehead and chin."*

At night, of course, when you'll be seen in artificial light, you can get away with more exotic colors, but always be sure that your blusher and lipstick are in the same family.

For myself, I prefer a creamy blusher. It's best for normal or dry skins and looks more natural on most faces though it may not last as well as powder. It comes in sticks, cakes, or jars, and you blend it on with your fingers or a sponge. Liquid colors and gels work well too.

Oily skins, however, are always better off with powder products. Makeup artist Kevyn Aucoin likes powder for everyone and puts it on with a soft brush (remember to tap off the excess first—Kevyn *blows* on his brush).

Cristina Ferrare likes to use *both* cream and powder blushers. She blends on a light cream rouge (pinky tones for her) and dusts a little powder blusher in the same shade over it to set it, making it last longer.

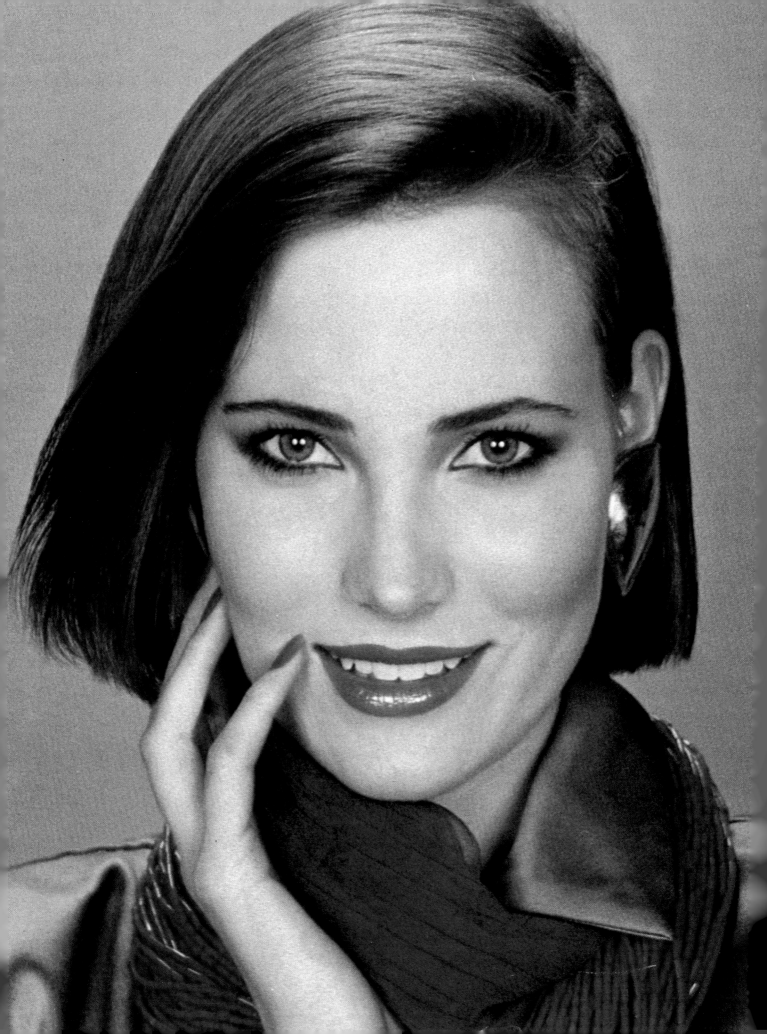

Another trick: Apply blusher in two stages, and you'll be less likely to overdo it. Put on a sheer coat, go about your business (maybe doing your eye makeup) for about ten minutes, and then take another look in a good light. Add more if you need it. Remove some with a tissue if you've gone overboard.

> **BLUSHER IS SMOOTHER,** *says Joyce Hartenstein, if you apply it in downward strokes in the same direction as the little facial hairs grow. I was strolling along a canal in Venice one day and spotted Joyce, an American girl on vacation. That's how she became a Ford model.*

WHERE THE BLUSHER GOES

To look healthy, natural, and twinkly, use blusher mainly on the "apples" of your cheeks, the part that rounds up when you smile, blending it into nothingness and out toward your hairline at the top of your ears.

Never apply blusher closer to your nose than the center of your eyes, because that makes your eyes look closer together. It also emphasizes a prominent nose.

Blusher looks great on other parts of your face, too, giving them a healthy glowing look if you use it carefully. Try a dot of blush on your chin and another on your forehead in the center just above your brow line. You might try another on the bridge of your nose. Cristina Ferrare likes it on her chin, forehead, and the tip of her nose. Blend, blend, blend.

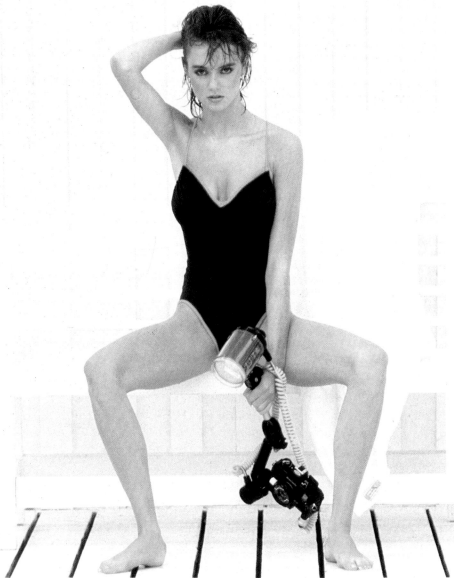

Vanessa Angel

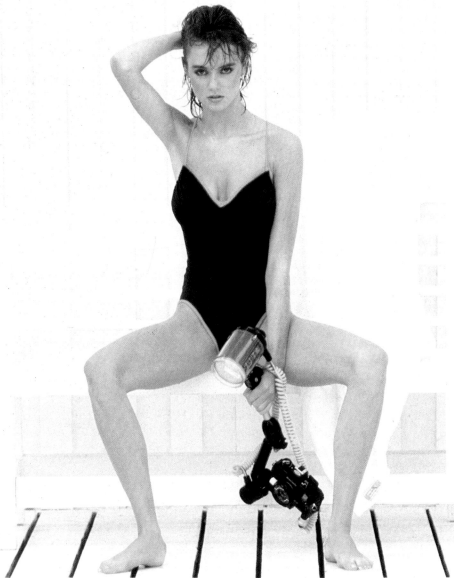

VANESSA ANGEL, *who has legendary English skin, uses powder blusher to narrow her wide cheeks. She blends light pink on her cheekbones and a darker shade in the hollow to give more definition and length to her face. To bring her high forehead down a little, she uses darker blush just along her hairline and on the temples.*

ANETTE STAI *uses blusher instead of base in winter. With her fingertips, she blends a brown-toned blush on her forehead, nose, around her hairline, the outer sides of her eyes, and between her eyes. "I just use a little," Anette says, "and it picks up my whole face."*

SHARI BELAFONTE, *whose skin is a beautiful golden tan color, likes blusher in an earthy tone all over her face, especially on her nose and the tip of her chin. "Just enough for a healthy glow," she says.*

VOILÀ! CHEEKBONES

Some women were born with gloriously high cheekbones. Some weren't. If you weren't, no reason to despair. To create the illusion of high cheekbones, you will need two shades of cheek color, one a little darker than the other. Feel your face and notice the diagonal hollows below your cheekbones. Apply the paler blusher on the bones themselves and continue it into the hairline above your ears; then apply the darker shade to the hollows, again blending outward. Blend the two together carefully. The darker area must look like a natural shadow. For even more emphasis, you can add a little frosted highlighter powder just along the top ridge of the bones. For evening, a tiny dab of silver or gold on the tip of the cheekbone looks fantastic.

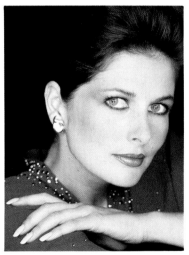

Cristina Ferrare

MORE SHAPING WITH BLUSHER

You can use blusher to shape other parts of your face, too. Use it high on your cheeks to make eyes look bigger and wider. Start at your cheekbones and blend up and out to your hairline as Maggie Fahy does. Dab some on your chin and the center of your forehead to slim a very round or square face. Conversely, to give width to a narrow face, concentrate the color toward the sides of your face, blending it lightly up alongside your brows. Never extend it below the end of your nose.

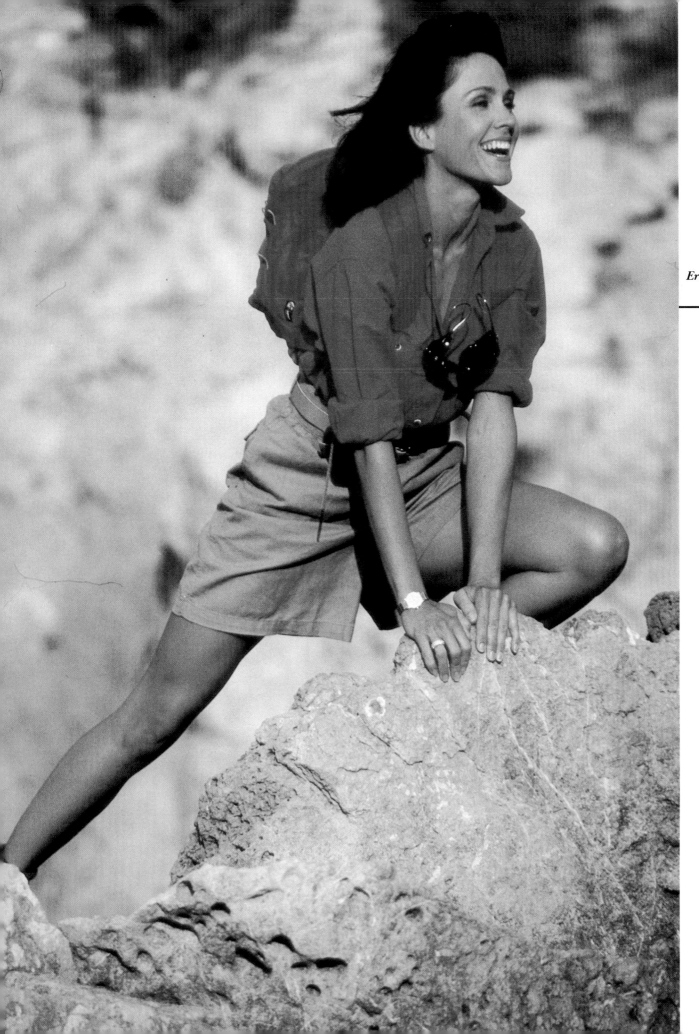

A LONG, THIN FACE *is what Erin Gray says she has (Erin's the spokeswoman for Bloomingdale's). She shortens her face with blusher, using a faint brownish shade right along her hairline. She also carries her soft cheekbone blusher right across the bridge of her nose. "Then I add little dabs on my chin and temples. It looks so healthy and glowing, especially when I have a little tan, and gives width to my face at the same time."*

PLAYING UP YOUR EYES

You'd be amazed if you saw some of our top models without their eye makeup. Eye makeup makes more difference in a woman's looks than any other cosmetic. It can turn a pretty girl into a fabulous beauty, and even our models who swear they don't wear any makeup when they're off duty will admit, when pressed, that they do wear mascara and eyeliner. That's because, unless they have naturally long, lush lashes, great coloring, enormous eyes, they—like you and me—can look drab.

Nothing changes a face faster than eye makeup. And nothing is misused as much, either. Most women use too little or too much, and I don't know which is worse. Too little looks washed out, and too much is aging and hard.

Here's the way we teach Ford models to make the most of their eyes. Let's start with eyebrows.

EYEBROW TAMING

Eyebrows are best when they look natural. Skinny little pencil-line eyebrows are out. Don't try to completely reshape what you're got, just im-

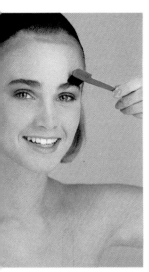

Joyce Hartenstein

prove on them. Follow their natural line and allow them to be slightly irregular. You want to look *real.* Brooke Shields, who for several years was one of Ford's child models, is a great example of how wonderful natural brows can be. She just removes the strays and stragglers and lets them be.

Always pluck from *underneath,* removing just enough to clean up the line. Be careful not to overpluck because once they're gone, they're usually gone. Along the top, remove only the strays. If your brows are too thick, pluck a few random hairs from the center to make them look softer. If they're too long and unruly, trim them a little with cuticle scissors.

For most women, the inner corners of the brows should begin above the inner corner of the eyes. The outer ends should be on a line from your nose to your temples. Hold a pencil at an angle from the bottom of your nose to the outer corners of your eyes. Where the pencil crosses your browbone is where your brows should stop. Though some women look wonderful with straight brows, for most of us a little arch opens up the eyes and makes them look bigger and more alive. Usually, the highest point of the arch should be directly over the outside edge of the iris (the colored part of the eye). Tweeze out *a few* hairs to give yourself an arch if you haven't got one. If you don't need an arch, forget it. Brooke Shields hasn't suffered from her straight-arrow brows. Juli Foster, whose brows are full and very dark, leaves hers alone except for the stragglers underneath.

If your eyes are too close-set, you can make them appear wider apart by starting the brows slightly beyond the inner corners of your eyes and extending them slightly beyond the outer corners. You can also arch them a little farther out. Not too much. Exaggeration will have the opposite effect from what you're looking for.

For eyes too widely spaced, do just the opposite. Start the brows closer to the bridge of your nose and end them slightly closer to the outer corners of your eyes. Arch them nearer to the center of your eyes. Only a little.

Tweeze brows before bed (it leaves you red for a while), just after a shower when your skin is soft, or hold a warm washcloth over them for a minute. Clean the area with alcohol on a cotton ball. Pull out just one hair at a time, using a gentle tug in the direction of growth. Do a little tweezing on one eye, then on the other, going back and forth. This way, you're less likely to end up with two different eyebrows.

ONE EYEBROW'S HIGHER *than the other in Debra Halley's case. So she tweezes the top of one brow and the bottom of the other to even them out.*

A current trend is to lighten overpowering eyebrows rather than tweeze them mercilessly. Professional bleaching can make them look much softer and less dominating. You can do it yourself, but I caution against it—I've seen too many orange eyebrows.

EYEBROW SHAPING

If your brows are skimpy or you've overdone the tweezer work, use an eyebrow pencil in a color that matches or is just slightly lighter than your natural color. Occasionally, a blonde whose brows are almost invisible requires a little darker shade. I like light brown with no red overtones. Auburn is for redheads. But never stray far from the color you've got. Never go very dark unless your hair is truly black, and then stay with deep brown or charcoal gray. Otherwise, you'll look ready to leap on stage and sing *Carmen*.

First, brush your brows with an eyebrow brush or an old toothbrush. Brush them up and out. This makes them look darker and fuller even without using added color. Shari Belafonte brushes hers straight up.

For really unruly brows, tame them with setting gel or hair spray. Jill Morris, for example, spritzes hair spray on an old toothbrush and brushes her eyebrows into shape. It makes them look fuller and keeps them under control. Rosemary McGrotha prefers petroleum jelly, and other models use lip gloss. Incidentally, Rosemary is one of three top Ford models from northern Florida.

To add color to your eyebrows, use powdered color, which is applied dry with a little slanted brush. Feather it on, using little short strokes and then brush everything back into shape.

To create a new shape, to fill in empty spots, or extend the brows, you'll do better with a pencil, a very sharp pencil. The lines you'll be drawing in must be as thin as real hairs. Simply stroke in hairs where you need them and go over everything with a brush. *Never* draw one single line across your brow.

WORKING WITH EYE SHADOW

Smudge shadow over your entire upper lids, blending it down to the lashes and up to your eyebrows, concentrating the color at the lashes and the outer corners and becoming paler towards the brows. Shadow under your lower lashes as well.

You can use the same shade for everything, simply applying it in different intensities. Or you can choose three different—but always compatible—colors: one for lids, one—darker—for the crease, and another—paler—for the area above. Plus highlighter, of course. For example, Maggie Fahy likes taupe on her lids, a darker taupe in the crease, a silver-gray highlighter and gray-brown surrounding her eyes. Nancy DeWeir tends to stick with tones of brown. Browns, taupes, plums, mushrooms, even burgundy, work well for almost everyone. Some models prefer grays. Experiment until you find your color.

A little highlighter paler than your lid shadow applied just under the browbones opens up your eyes and creates space. Always keep it faint and almost undetectable especially during the day. At night, you can be more dramatic.

LINING YOUR EYES

Surrounding your eyes with color makes your lashes look thicker and your eyes bigger and brighter. It gives pale eyes definition and makes dark eyes more impressive. Use a soft eyeliner pencil or a powder applied with a small brush, drawing a thick line as close as possible to the roots of your lashes. Try holding the lids slightly taut with one hand while you work with the other. This gives you a smoother surface to draw on. If your hand is wobbly, rest the heel on your cheek.

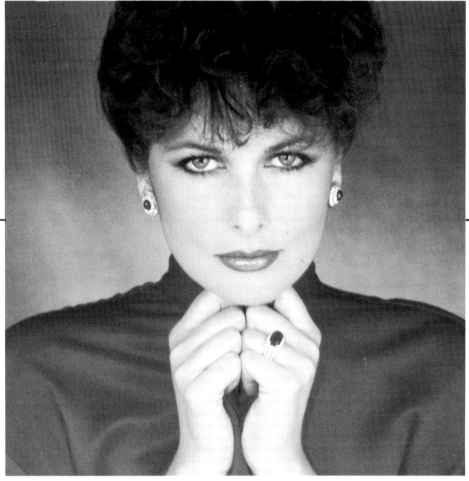

Cristina Ferrare

"DON'T LEAVE SPACE *between the lash line and the eyeliner," advises Cristina Ferrare. She likes charcoal gray or sable brown eye shadow powder applied with a soft brush dipped in water, says it gives a softer line than pencil.*

Line both lids, concentrating the color toward the outer ends of the eyes (exception: see below for wide-spaced eyes). Most women look best with liner only on the outer two thirds of the eyes. If your eyes are too close together, just line the outer halves.

Since the purpose of eyeliner is to make your lashes look lush and your eyes stand out—not to look like a raccoon—you must now smudge the line so it's soft and shadowy. Do it with your fingertip, a spongetip applicator, or a Q-tip. Hard lines are aging. Barbara Neumann makes a thick line toward the outer corners, using black shadow and a slanted brush. Smudged, it opens up her eyes. Cheryl Tiegs draws a soft line *under* her eyes to lift the outer corners. Juli Foster likes eyeliner all along the top edge of the eyes and just a touch on the lower lids. Cristina Ferrare lines hers all around.

"FOR NARROW EYES *like mine,"*
says Carrie Peterson, "eyeliner
gives them wonderful definition and
the illusion of more width. I use a
dark pencil and blend it with a Q-
tip."

Unless you're a natural beauty and are deft with the tools, it's best to skip the blacks and deep browns. At least, be sure to smudge them till they are truly soft. Try the lighter browns, smokey grays, cinnamons, the earthy tones. And as for color eyeliners, forget it. I've never liked them, and I never will. Except for photography when exaggeration is needed or under dim lights on a big night, it looks cheap.

ROSEMARY McGROTHA *puts her*
liner on in dots, *then blends all the*
dots together into a soft smudge.
She finds the color easier to control
that way. Maybe you will, too.

Rimming the *insides* of your eyes gives an intense and sultry look. Cristina Ferrare always uses this technique to make her dark eyes even more out-standing, but warns against it if your eyes are small because it closes them up. Kirsten Allen likes a dark blue line to make her blue eyes stand out more. Vibeke lines hers just inside her lashes with black or gray or some-times purple. "It sets off my eyes and makes the whites look whiter. Pull the lower lid down and your upper lid up with one hand and run a very soft pencil just on the dry edge." Shari Belafonte, who wears little makeup off-stage—she's in a TV series and stars in some fantastic Calvin Klein jeans ads and commercials—always lines inside her lashes with a soft smudge-proof black liner and swears it makes her eyes look much bigger.

SPOT REMOVER: *To remove makeup mistakes, keep some Q-tips handy. Dip one in makeup remover or cleansing lotion (don't use oil) and wipe off the errant color.*

LUSH LASHES

Make sure your lashes are bone-dry and oil-free. Then curl them. They will seem much thicker and longer. Curl them a couple of times, if necessary—some models with stiff straight lashes do it three or even four times.

DON'T *EVER* CURL YOUR LASHES *after you've put on your mascara, insists Maggie Fahy, who appears in so many TV commercials that it's almost impossible to keep track of her. "I did that once on location, and I pulled out most of the lashes on one eye. Don't do it in a moving car, either! One pothole and you're in big trouble!"*

Mascara in a wand is the easiest to use, though cake mascara applied with water and a brush is the favorite of many makeup artists because it doesn't clump as easily. I don't believe in anything but black mascara. If you're looking for longer lashes, try one of those lash builders. Used adeptly it works, but many models complain that those little fibers get in their eyes or fall off onto their cheekbones.

An alternative to this is powdering your lashes. The mascara will go on thicker and last longer. Apply mascara first to your bottom lashes, then the top. Cover from base to tip with sweeping strokes. If the color tends to clump, use the wand vertically, separating the hairs. Coat both sides of both sets of lashes. (If you don't like what mascara on your bottom lashes does for your eyes, just apply it to the top.)

Two coats of mascara are the minimum. Let the lashes dry in between and comb them with a tiny lash comb or a clean, dry mascara brush. Powder again before a new application.

THREE OR EVEN FOUR COATS *of mascara are routine for Vibeke because her lashes are straight and not very luxurious. She curls them, dabs powder on them, then goes at them with the black mascara.*

Some mascaras are waterproof. These are very hard to remove, even with special removers, and they're hard on your lashes as a result. Save them for summer when you're in and out of water. Or you can have your lashes dyed professionally.

INSTEAD OF MASCARA, *"Face of the '80s" winner Anette Stai often dabs her eyelashes with night cream. It makes them look darker and lubricates them at the same time. "My lashes tend to get very dry when I use mascara constantly," Anette states.*

Fill in any sparse spaces with dark eyeliner, giving the illusion of lashes and lushness.

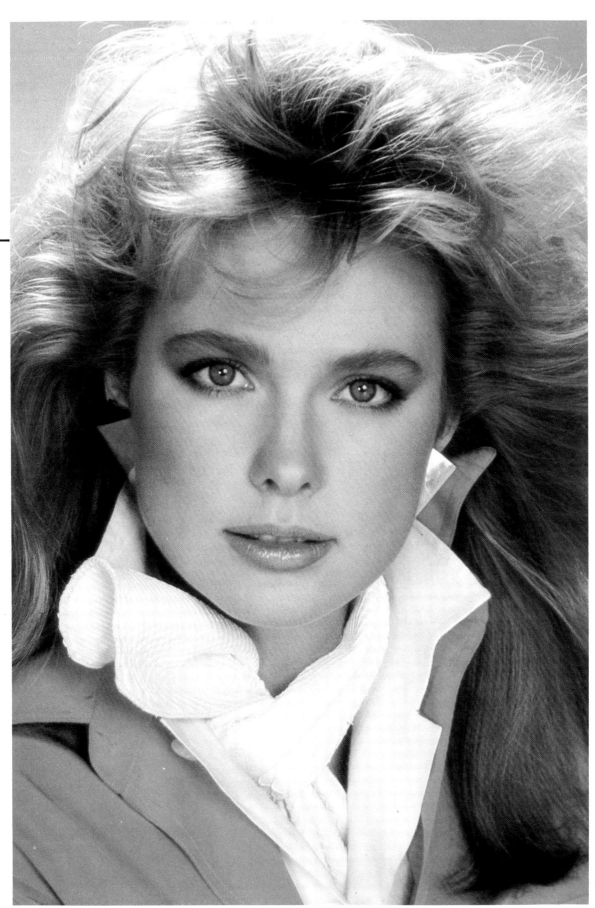

Nancy DeWeir

TAKING MASCARA OFF

Water-based mascara is no problem to remove. It comes off along with your other makeup and dirt when you wash your face or cleanse with creams or lotions. For waterproof or oil-based mascara, however, you need eye makeup remover or oil to dissolve it. Dampen a cotton ball with the remover, close your eyes, and wipe the cotton down your lashes, under which you have placed some tissue, then across the lids. Don't rub.

OPTICAL ILLUSIONS: TIPS FROM THE PROFESSIONALS

If your eyes aren't perfect, here's what you can do.

• *Small Eyes:* Concentrate shadow on the outer two-thirds of your eyes. Apply a pale neutral shadow all over your entire upper lids, then deepen the tone from the lashline to the crease, and go even darker along the crease itself. Line both lids with a dark pencil starting about a third of the way from your inner corners, smudging it up and out beyond the outer corners on top. Finish with at least two coats of black mascara.

TO MAKE HER EYES BIGGER,
Kathryn Redding uses a lash curler first, then lines her eyes with dark brown or rust to open them up. "Black's much too harsh for me." Then she smudges the line so it seems like a dark shadow. She keeps her eye shadow very light, uses browns, rusts, and pinks. And wears pale lipstick so her eyes stand out more and her mouth looks generous. And, oh yes, two coats of brown mascara.

• *Close-set Eyes:* Keep the shadow near your nose very light and intensify the color in an outward sweep toward the ends of your eyebrows. Apply highlighter just under your browbone and in the dark recesses near your nose. Line the outer two-thirds of the eyes with dark eyeliner, extending it slightly beyond the corners and smudging until the line is soft. Concentrate mascara on the outer lashes. Extend the ends of your eyebrows just slightly.

• *Wide-spaced Eyes:* Blend the shadow more intensely toward your nose. Line your entire eyes with smudged pencil. Draw your eyebrows slightly closer over your nose and end them just inside the ends of your eyes.

WIDE-EYED KERSTIN MARIE, *Swedish, raised in Australia, draws shadow across the entire lid but makes sure it's not too dark at the outer ends, and stops short of the corners.*

• *Deep-set Eyes:* Stay with paler shadows on the lids, ending the color just above the crease. Use a neutral shade above the crease. Do not highlight the browbone. Line the outer halves of both lids, widening the line as you go, and smudge.

STAR OF MANY HALSTON FASH-ION SHOWS, *Chris Royer has deep-set eyes, so she never uses strong eye colors. Instead, she likes a very pale silvered brown on her lids and a cinnamon eyeliner. She adds a dot of highlighter right in the middle of her top lid just above the iris.*

• ***Bulging Lids:*** Keep your shadow quite dark, especially near the lashes. Never use shiny colors.

• ***Round Saucer Eyes:*** Concentrate the color at the outer corners. Bring it down under the lower lashes at the outside corners. Line the inside rims of your upper lids and the outside half of the lower lids.

"DOWNWARD HALFMOONS" *is how Glynnis Jones describes her eyes. She brings them up at the ends by using brown shadow blended into a little upward triangle just above the outer corners of her eyes.*

TO EMPHASIZE HER ALMOND EYES, *Vanessa Angel intensifies the color at the upper corners. She likes grays and browns for real life, purples and pinks for photography. The outer two-thirds of her eyes are lined with smudged pencil.*

MOUTH MAGIC

One of the miracles you can perform with makeup is a total redesign of your mouth. Is it too thin, too full, crooked, uneven, droopy, too peaked, no corners? Does it need to be played up or played down? Ford models make the most of theirs.

Don't always wear the same color lipstick. Experiment with colors and change them to suit what you're wearing. Models carry a complete wardrobe of lipsticks, maybe 30 or 40. That's going a little far, but give yourself a choice of at least 10 or 15 shades. Gloss is wonderful, too, though too much makes some women look hard.

If there's one feature that characterizes the newer, younger models today, it's their big mouths! Everyone's looking for full and sensuous lips. Well, that's great if you have them—you can play them up. But if you don't, you can fake it amazingly well. You can use the subtle tricks models who don't have big mouths use to make theirs look bigger. Or you can, as many of them do, simply make the most of what you've got. Ty Hendrick, for example, says she's got a small mouth and likes it just the way it is. Erin Gray, who's not only the spokeswoman for Bloomingdale's but is starring in a TV series, obviously hasn't suffered from the lack of lush lips. Neither has Cheryl Tiegs.

Start your mouth makeup with the lip primer or fixer if your lipstick tends to run. Choose a soft lipliner pencil the same color or just slightly darker than your lipstick. Outline your mouth, from the center of each lip out. Keep your mouth relaxed and slightly open, your elbow down or resting on a table. Hold the lipliner as you would a pencil, resting your little finger against your cheek to steady your hand. If you hold your mouth taut with two fingers of your other hand, you'll get a smooth surface to work on.

Now fill in your mouth with the pencil. This provides a good base for the lipstick, makes it last. Stroke your lipstick with a lipbrush and apply the color over your entire mouth, starting at the centers of the lips. Be sure you cover the lipliner, too. No obvious lines or demarcations allowed.

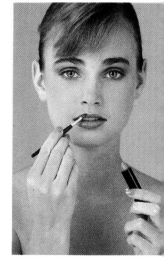

Joyce Hartenstein

Blot your lips with a tissue. No, it's not outdated. It helps hold it longer and mattes the color.

If you like shine, finish with lip gloss. A little dab of gloss right in the middle of the bottom lip gives a nice dewy effect.

"IF YOU WANT YOUR EYES *to really sparkle, use lots of gloss on your lips. It seems to reflect."* That's a piece of advice from Anette Stai.

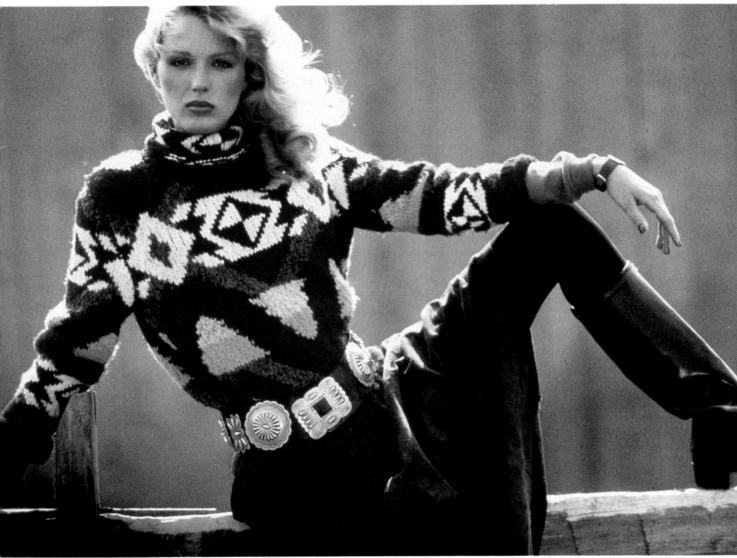

Kim Charlton

LIP TRICKS

• ***To Make Thin Lips Look Fuller:*** Draw the line around your mouth *just outside* your natural lipline, ending just short of each corner. Go over the line and the rest of your mouth with lipstick, using a light bright color. Lighter shades are best for a thin mouth because they make it look less defined. Dark colors make it look thinner and sharper. Highlight the middle of both lips with gloss.

   "Don't be afraid to enlarge your mouth," says Kim Charlton. "You simply draw it a little larger. I always do that for photography and sometimes when I go out at night." Alda Balestra also likes her mouth to seem bigger than life. An artist with the lipliner, she designs the shape she likes, fills in with lipstick, then blots, applies more lipstick, blots again. "If you're careful," she says, "it really looks real."

• ***To Make Full Lips Look Thinner:*** Since full mouths are more than acceptable today, I don't think many women should try to slim theirs down.

But if yours is truly out of proportion, draw the lipline just *inside* the natural perimeters of your mouth, ending just short of each corner. Fill in with a medium color. Don't use shine.

Jacki Adams has a wide, generous mouth, just the kind the fashion magazines yearn to find in a model, but she doesn't want her mouth to dominate her face too much. "My mouth has been an asset in my work," she says, "but I don't want to make it ridiculous. You need a harmony, a balance, so I don't overemphasize it. On the other hand, you can't be afraid of what's on your face and try to change it too much." Jacki follows the exact shape of her mouth with lipliner and prefers lipstick in midtone or pale sheer tones, perhaps corally pink, with no frost or shine.

More Lip Tricks

• **To Play Up Full Lips:** Color the lower lip a little lighter than the top, then add some shine to it.

GLYNNIS JONES *has a nice, full mouth, just what we look for today. To make it seem even poutier, she uses light lipstick colors.*

"MY MOST PROMINENT FEATURE *is my mouth," says Kathryn Redding. (Well, it's* one *of her prominent features. Another is her flaming red hair.) "Makeup artists use light lipstick to make my lips look even larger. And they smudge the lipliner so it doesn't have a sharp edge."*

• *If You Just Want a Little Color:* Apply lipstick, let it set, and wipe it off. Or put the color on with your finger. Or gloss your lips, then rub them with lipstick.

> **CHERYL TIEGS,** *whose mouth is a bit thin, usually extends her lipstick just a fraction beyond her natural lipline.*

• *If One Lip Is Too Thin,* the other comparatively full, draw the lipliner along the outer edge of the thin lip, the inner edge of the full lip. Sharpen the lipliner first, says Nina Renshaw.

> **"MY BOTTOM LIP IS FULLER THAN THE TOP,"** *says Vanessa Angel. She uses a slightly paler shade on the thinner top and dots a dark spot right in the middle of the lower lip to make it look smaller.*

• *Droopy Mouth:* If the corners of your mouth turn down, be sure you've put on your base and powder, then draw the corners just a tiny bit upwards, filling in with lipstick. Add gloss in the middle of your upper lip.

• *Overly Long Mouth:* Outline lips with lipliner and stop just short of the outer corners. Use a neutral beigey lipstick, with a little darker tone toward the outside.

"MY LIPS ARE CROOKED." *That's Maggie Fahy talking. To straighten them out she uses a pale beigey-pink skin-tone lipliner and blocks out the very edge of the fuller side, then applies her lipstick with a brush inside that line. Matte powder goes on top.*

ERIN GRAY'S REDESIGN: *Erin's mouth has a cupid's bow that comes to little peaks in the center, and her upper lip ends before it reaches the corners of her mouth. "So I correct it," she says, "by rounding the peak just a little and drawing in the ends of my upper lip where it disappears. Just enough to be undetectable. Then I fill everything in with a very soft color. No dark colors—the darker the lipstick, the tighter your lips look."*

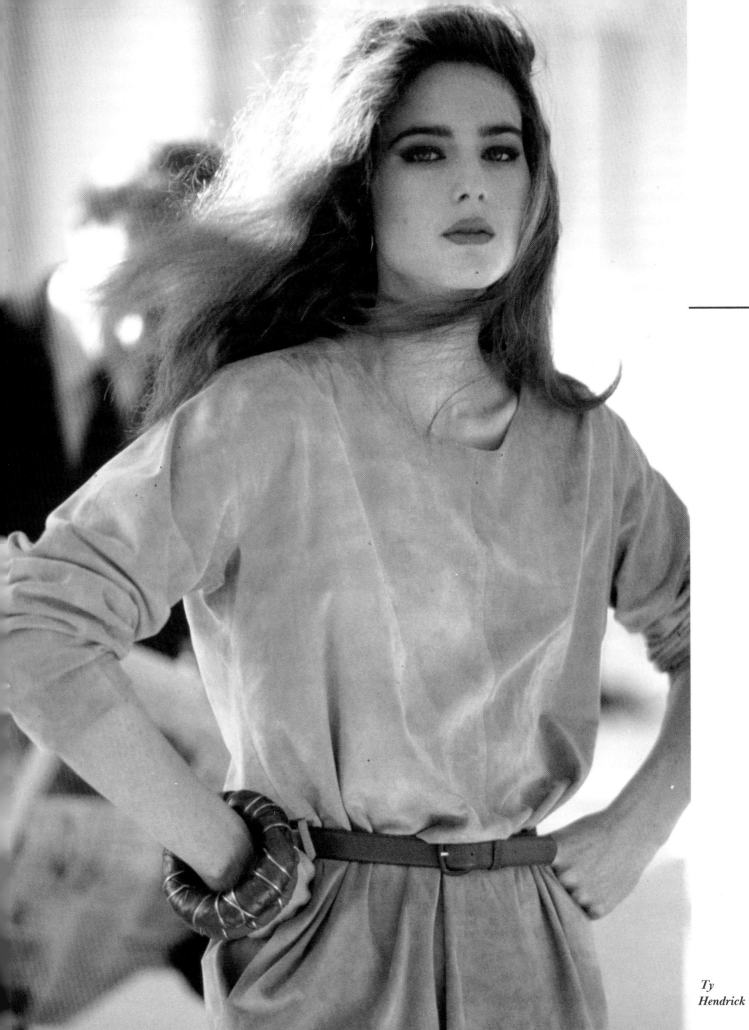

3

HOW TO HAVE SUPER HAIR

There isn't a woman alive who doesn't think she has a hair problem, including most of the models you see swinging their lustrous locks in all those television commercials. Nobody's satisfied with her own hair—it's always too straight or too curly, too dry, too oily, too thin, too something that makes her miserable. I am convinced women spend more time, money, and effort trying to change their hair than anything else. They can do it, too, if they know what our models know.

No matter what kind of hair you have, you can make it *look* wonderful. Many of our best models are proof of that statement, and I've asked them, as well as some of the top hair stylists who work with us, to share their secrets so you can profit from them too.

Some people do have naturally great hair. They were *born* with it. In the modeling business, great hair is the equivalent of owning a share of the United States Government Mint. The companies making hair-care products conduct a constant search for models with wonderful hair for their commercials and magazine ads, and the girls lucky enough to have it are always busy. We can't find enough time in their schedules for all their bookings.

All Ford models have reasonably good hair because we wouldn't have chosen them if they didn't, but—except for those fortunate few with the naturally great hair—models have their problems, too. They have simply learned to deal with them and keep their hair healthy, gleaming, and fashionably cut. A model whose hair won't cooperate is soon looking for other work.

One of the first concerns on a new model's agenda is a detailed discussion of her hair and what should be done with it. Almost always, she has arrived on our premises with a *lot* of hair, sometimes reaching right down to the middle of her back (and spends much of her time during our initial interviews stroking it!). Because long, long hair is hopelessly out of fashion today and a model must be on top of the trends, it must come off. Persuading a new model to have it cut, however, is one of the hardest jobs we have.

That's been true since we first started in business. I remember when Jean Patchett, the first model we ever made into a star, walked through our door. She sat there, her long hair streaming down her back, and I told her, "You'll have to cut it." "I can't!" she cried. "This is *me!*" But off it came—an inch at a time, I'll admit—until finally it was just right for one of the most successful careers ever.

After we decide what should be done for a new model's hair, she is sent to one of New York's best hairdressers for styling and perhaps some color. It's astonishing, even to us, what a difference the right hair cut or a slight color change can make. It can turn a hopeful into a star. Sometimes, of course, we don't get it right the first time around. I remember one girl at our affiliate agency in Milan. We thought she was wonderful, but she got only occasional bookings until her hair was cut in a radical new style. Almost immediately, her bookers couldn't keep up with the demands for her time.

Models today are spoiled. Most clients provide professional hairdressers in the studio or on location to style their hair, so usually a clean head of manageable hair is all that's required. But that's not always the case. Especially for runway work or catalogue photography, models must know how to set their own hair or at least give it direction. So they travel with a set of hot rollers, perhaps a curling iron, some mousse, gel, hair spray, clips, and can do a creditable job in short order.

> **JENNIFER BERRINGTON,** *who specializes in catalogue work and therefore usually styles her own hair, carries a butane curling iron in her bag. "It's changed my life," she says. "It's light and cordless, fills up like a cigarette lighter. I turn the ends under and my bangs back, and I'm ready to go." She also trims the ends regularly to get rid of the split ends caused by the constant heat.*

START WITH THE BASICS

Maybe you're not going to turn your hair into dollars like the industry's top hair models, but you can certainly turn it into one of your major assets. That means you must know the basics of hair fitness. Style today is seldom much more than an excellent cut and only a minor amount of setting or direction, so keeping your hair healthy and fit is more important than it ever was before.

Healthy, fit, beautiful hair doesn't just happen. Even for those few lucky people with naturally great hair, it doesn't last without care. As our famous cover girl Cheryl Tiegs once said, "You can't neglect yourself and then hope to turn into Cinderella." Just like good skin, good hair requires a healthy diet, regular exercise, enough sleep, and the right beauty routines.

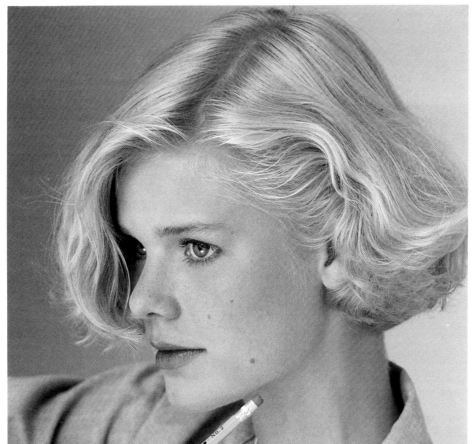

Anna Magnusson

SECRETS OF A GOOD SHAMPOO

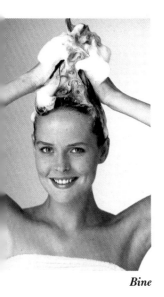

Bine

You don't have to wash your hair every day unless it's very oily or you work in a coal mine. Two or three times a week is usually sufficient. Models, of course, are so lacquered and sprayed all day long that the first thing most of them do when they get home is remove their makeup and wash their hair. But even they often let it go longer when they can, because overwashing is so drying.

Eva Voorhis, for example, alternates shampoos with wetting and conditioning her hair in the shower. Brooke Shields, the first child model we ever signed at the agency, recently went public with the information that she washes hers every other day. Susan Hess, who likes everything natural, lets hers go four or five days, because, she says, it's dry and washing it takes the body out. "You're just removing your own natural oil and then putting it back in." She rinses with warm water and brushes her scalp with a soft brush.

> **SUPER-SHORT HAIR** *is what Donna Stia is wearing these days, and she can't wash it every day or it lies flat to her head. Donna, who does mostly fashion photography and is constantly booked all over the world, has blond hair that is super-fine as well as supershort. "I let it go for a couple of days so I don't have to gunk it up with products to get volume. I just give it a quick rinse with warm water, comb it in place, and let it dry."*

Before shampooing, give your scalp a good massage with your fingertips, pressing firmly and moving in little circles so your scalp moves with your fingers.

Choose a mild shampoo designed for your kind of hair. Today that's no problem—all shampoos are clearly labeled. Wet your head with warm water, apply a little shampoo, and massage it lightly into your hair, concentrating on the scalp and hairline.

Don't use your fingernails, though you may want to scrub gently with one of those little soft scalp brushes. Cheri La Rocque always uses one. (Discovered while playing badminton in her high-school gym class, Cheri promptly made the cover of *Seventeen*. When we saw it, I arranged to meet her on one of my trips to California. Her mother, she says, convinced her to come to New York one summer to try modeling. She came, and she stayed.)

Rinse your hair thoroughly, then rinse some more to be sure all the shampoo is out, especially if you have coarse hair which is very absorbent. Leftover residue can take the gloss right out.

One sudsing is plenty. Two latherings tend to remove too much natural oil. If you can stand it, give your hair a final rinse with cold water for extra shine.

WILLOW BAY, *whose face you've learned to love in the Estée Lauder ads, washes her thin, fine, blunt-cut hair at least once a day, sometimes twice, with a very mild camomile-and-oatmeal shampoo. Then she gives it a final rinse with club soda. Guaranteed to promote a shine, she says.*

Another way to help remove shampoo residue is a next-to-final rinse with diluted vinegar. That's how it's done by **ALDA BALESTRA,** *our model from northern Italy who is under contract to L'Oréal and in constant demand as well for runway shows in every fashion capital of the world.*

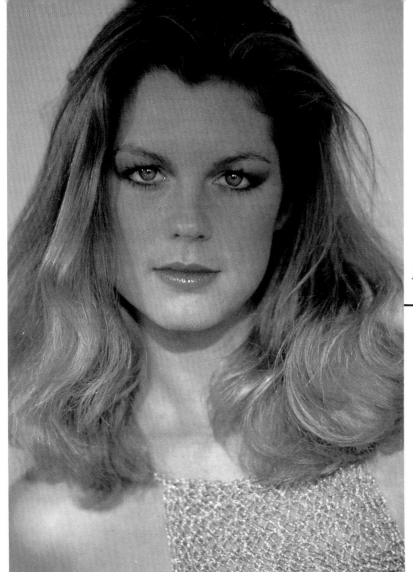

Donna Sexton

Kim Charlton

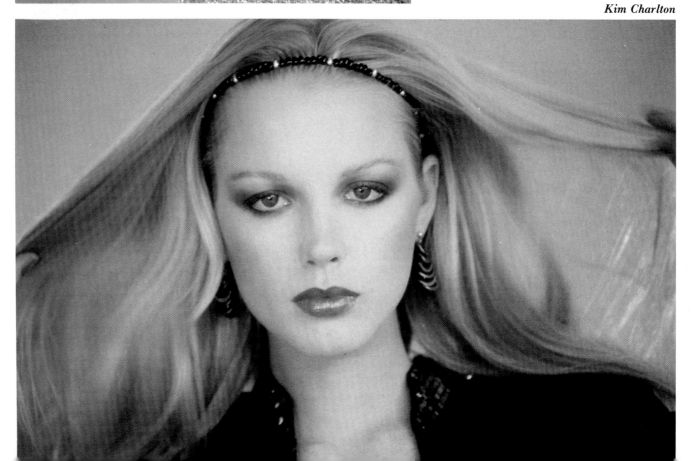

CONDITIONING: THE VITAL STEP (FOR MOST OF US)

If your hair is dry, and especially if it's been permed or colored, you probably need an instant conditioner every time you wash your hair. If it's oily, you may need conditioner on the ends.

After you've shampooed your hair, work in a little conditioner (not much, warns Kim Lepine, one of the hair stylists we send new models to for styling, unless your hair is coarse, frizzy, or truly damaged, or you'll end up with hair that's too soft to manage). Leave it in for about a minute and rinse out thoroughly. The purpose of conditioner is to coat the hair, filling in the rough spots, making it smoother, thicker, and shinier. It also prevents tangling, controls flyaway hair, reduces static electricity, adds body, seals in moisture.

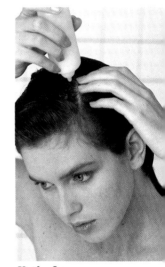

Kathy Law

> **MAURA, THE CLINIQUE GIRL** *who lives an outdoor California life, has thick, curly, dark blond hair to which she does as little as possible. If you had her hair, you'd do the same. She never perms it or blow-dries it, brushes it minimally, wears a hat in the sun—all this to keep it virginal and healthy. She uses conditioner only on the very ends where it tends to be dry.*

Many models don't use conditioner at all, or only occasionally. It makes their hair too limp. Kerstin Marie, for example, skips it on working days or her hair is unmanageable. Juli Foster uses it only once a week at night. She washes her hair, applies the conditioner, goes to bed, lets it work while she sleeps, rinses it out in the morning. And Linda Tonge, one of the few models who admits to having an oily scalp, washes her hair every day but doesn't use conditioner because it makes her hair droopy.

What's best for you? The only way to find out is by trial and error. Just like everybody else, you must experiment to see how your hair responds.

About once a week, give your hair a heavy-duty intensive conditioning treatment if your hair is dry or damaged. Directions differ, so follow those on the package. Most conditioners are applied to wet hair, left on for 15 minutes to an hour, rinsed out. This kind of conditioner is creamy or oily and replaces the lubricants and moisture you are missing. Obviously, if your hair is oily, you don't need it. If your hair is "normal" (neither dry nor oily), you don't need it, either.

AFTER A DAY AT THE BEACH,
Sarah Stimson, who was signed up as a Ford model the same day she walked into the agency for an interview, rinses her hair, conditions it and doesn't wash it out until the next morning. "Sometimes I use lanolin instead," she says, "because my hair gets so dry."

DO-IT-YOURSELF OIL TREATMENTS

An astounding number of models use oil as an occasional alternative to deep conditioning. If you have excessively dry hair, split ends, or your hair's been overprocessed by perms or coloring, try it.

Kathryn Redding, who describes her glorious red hair as "just like horse-hair" (very dry and very coarse), heats up olive oil or safflower oil every two weeks, puts it in her hair for half an hour. Clotilde, the girl with the thick shiny dark hair in the Ralph Lauren ads, rubs olive oil into the dry ends only. Then she wears two tight braids for a couple of days before loosening them and giving her hair a good shampoo. "My hair drinks the oil up," she says.

Evelyn Kuhn pulls a plastic bag over her olive-oiled hair and lets it soak for a few hours. Sometimes she mixes in a little vinegar too, then washes it all out with hot water and baby shampoo. And Eva Johansson spends entire weekends walking around with baby oil in her blond hair. She says baby oil

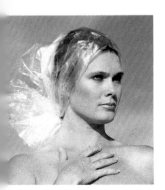

Barbara Neumann

is easier to remove than olive oil. According to stylist Kim Lepine, almond oil washes out best. Mayonnaise is, of course, an excellent oil treatment for dry hair.

Rosemary McGrotha, a top hair model whose long, dark brown hair gets dry from the hazards of the business, has her own recipe for a hair conditioner: One egg yolk, the contents of a vitamin E capsule, two tablespoons of virgin olive oil. Apply for half an hour twice a month. Rosemary is one of the models we signed up within minutes of meeting her. From Tallahassee, Florida, she came to New York, walked into the agency, and that was that.

DO-IT-YOURSELF CONDITIONER

concocted by Christie Brinkley: Mix a little mashed avocado with coconut milk (you can buy it in health-food stores). Comb it through your hair, let it sit there for about ten minutes, and rinse out.

Oil works best with a plastic bag or some plastic wrap on your head. Heat helps, too, so sit under a dryer or a heat lamp or go outside when the sun's shining.

Let me warn you: Oil may be hard to get out. You'll need at least a double shampoo and a lot of hot water. Brunettes needn't be too concerned, but blonds sometimes get a slight darkening effect that lasts a couple of shampoos.

DRYING THE GENTLE WAY

Blot your hair with a towel, then wrap the towel around your head for a few minutes to soak up some more water. Towel dry gently. Wet hair is much more fragile than dry and can be damaged by overenthusiasm. Best to let it dry in the air and push it into place with your fingers. Brush gently—wet hair doesn't have much elasticity and breaks easily. Instead, use a wide-toothed comb with round teeth, combing the ends first, then working up to

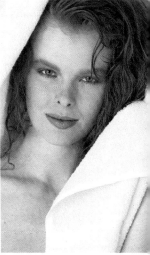

Kathryn Redding

the scalp. If you suffer from tangles, the conditioner should alleviate the situation. The time to brush is after your hair is dry, but never for the traditional 100 strokes. Brush only enough to distribute oil and smooth the hair, very gently and slowly.

If you can let your hair dry naturally, great. If you need to blow dry, allow your hair to dry in the air until it's just damp and then use the dryer. To minimize heat damage, don't hold the blower too close to your head, and keep it moving. When it is almost dry, turn it to a cooler setting. Never blow hair after it is completely dry unless you're looking for split ends and straw hair.

HOW TO GET VOLUME

Hair that lies down flat on your head is, no doubt, the Number One hair affliction for most women. In fact, hair stylist Bruno Demetrio of Le Salon, who is one of the experts to whom we send new models, says, "Ninety percent of the women I see, including all the models who are my clients, *hate* flat hair. They want *volume!*" What's more, they want it with little effort—in and out of the shower looking great. Nobody goes to bed with a headful of rollers anymore.

If you don't have natural volume, you can get it. There have been so many scientific breakthroughs and new styling techniques developed in the last few years that nobody has to live with the limp hair she was born with.

Models, who rarely have perms (except for the special kinds we'll talk about later) because their hair must remain totally adaptable, get volume with good haircuts, mousses, and gels and sculpting lotions, plus some simple drying techniques designed to produce body and lift.

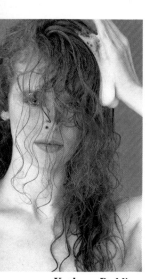

Kathryn Redding

Mousses, gels and sculpting lotions are actually strong setting lotions that don't make your hair sticky or stiff and dry very quickly. Mousse works on wet or dry hair and can make it more manageable and full. Squirt a blob about the size of an egg into your hand, rub it between your palms, and work it through your hair from the roots outward to the ends. Then place the hair with your hands or a comb, or run your fingers through it for a lift. You can even make waves by forming them and holding them in place with long clips until dry. Or use the mousse only in strategic areas—for lift at your bangs, for example—if that's all you need.

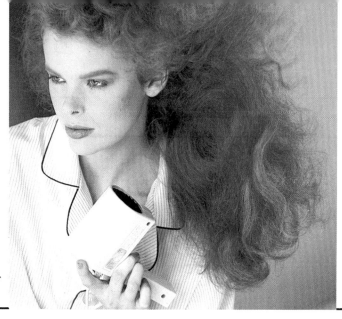

Kathryn Redding

KERSTIN MARIE, *who is Swedish but grew up in Australia, is one model who's been truly saved by mousse. She wets her pale blond hair, sprays mousse on the roots, lets it dry with her head upside down. In a hurry, she uses sculpting lotion on dry hair the same way. She gets more fullness, too, by having her limp hair cut a little shorter in the underneath layers.*

UP IN FRONT: *Here's how Donna Stia gets the lift she likes in the front of her short superfine hair. She combs it in place with mousse or sculpting lotion, ties a kerchief around her head about two inches back from the hairline. She pushes the kerchief forward, puffing up the front of her hair with it, and lets it dry. You can do the same thing with a hair band. Or try lifting the top and sides with two- or three-inch combs.*

Gel usually works best for short hair because it's relatively heavy. It makes hair look thicker and full of body. It can be used to give volume or direction or take curl out of the hair. Take a little in your palm (about the size of a nickel), rub your hands together to distribute it, and slick it through damp hair. Blow dry, directing the hair with fingers or a round brush, or push the hair into the shape you want and let it dry by itself.

You can use it just at the hairline for volume in front, as Juli Foster does. Apply the gel, then lift with your fingers. Or sleek your hair down as Kirsten Allen, who flies to New York to work for a few days a month bringing her 12th-grade homework with her, does to pin her short hair back from her face.

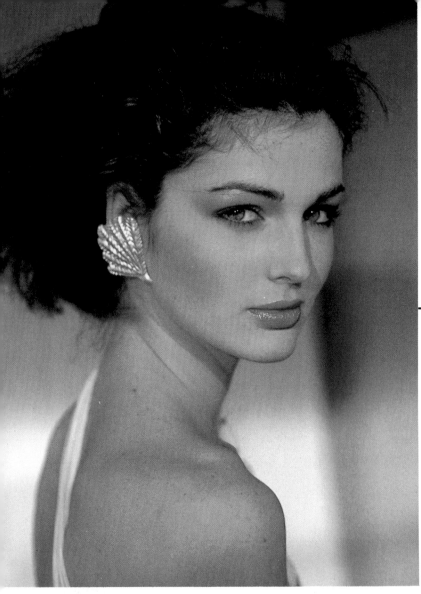

Eva Voorhis

MORE VOLUME TRICKS FROM FORD MODELS

- Blow dry your hair upside down, the way Cheryl Tiegs does.

- Finger-fluff it from roots to ends as it dries. Toss it back when it's almost totally dry. Some models apply gel or mousse on the underside of the hair first.

SPOT WELDING: *Another use for the new gels and lotions is to anchor a particular section of hair. Jill Morris sprays her hairbrush with sculpting lotion and then brushes the hair into place. Jill is known for her lithe, lean body, delicate features, and total reliability.*

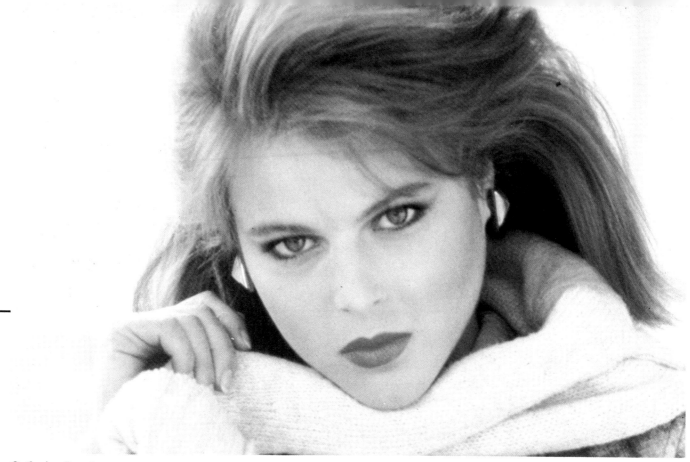

Catherine Oxenberg

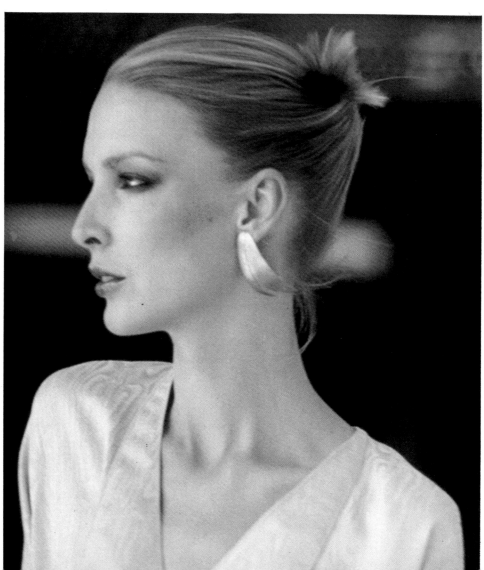

Karen Bjornson

- Quick pickup: To add lift during the day, mist your hair lightly, then with sculpting lotion on your palms slide your fingers into your hair and lift and shape.

- The simplest hair-styling, volume-producing method comes from Anette Stai: She holds the back of her wet head in front of a fan and brushes it dry! Another lucky one with great hair, Anette's blunt-cut blond hair is strong and healthy and thick.

PERM POINTERS

Permanents are famous for saving the sanity of limp-haired women. They can change your life, take the anxiety out of a damp day, let you wake up in the morning looking presentable. Perms, which used to produce a lot of frizz and frequent heartache, have been perfected to give you just what you want—controlled curls or waves, or only volume, body, and manageability.

Perms come out best on virginal and healthy hair, so it's smart not to repeat the process too frequently. It's best to let your hair grow out before getting another. You can, however, perm *parts* of your hair—the top, for example, where it's gone flat.

Direction or style is not a perm's function. It merely provides wave, a little or a lot, which you must then take charge of. If you like total curl, towel dry and let your hair dry as is, fluffing it up with a hair pick. Or you can blow it dry on low heat, style it with your fingers or a vent brush. Some prefer to mold their perms with mousse or gel, placing it, rolling it, or smoothing it with their hands or a brush. Sometimes a few strategically placed rollers in almost-dry hair are all you need.

Always get a perm at least a couple of weeks before coloring. If you get the color first, the chemicals used in the permanenting process may change it into a color you hadn't planned on.

In addition to the usual curly/wavy perm and the body wave (designed specifically for volume rather than curl and therefore produced on larger rods), there are a number of other varieties available today.

The "root perm" is a technique where only an inch or so of the hair at the roots is rolled and processed. This lifts the hair gently and makes it look fuller and thicker, leaving the top hair smooth.

The "reverse perm" gives a soft lift just around the face, redirecting the hair away from the face. Or it can be used to relax too much curl.

An "under perm" is similar to a root perm. It adds volume by perming only the underlayers, fluffing them up to greater fullness, but again, the top hair is untouched.

A "spot wave" will produce volume or body and/or curl in a specific area only, wherever you need help. The top is the usual location for a spot wave.

PERM CARE

Perms are drying. And they make your hair more fragile, just as any chemical process does. Use a shampoo specifically made for processed hair and be sure to apply an instant conditioner after every wash and a deep conditioner once a week to restore some of the lost moisture.

Always wait at least 48 hours after getting a perm before washing your hair, to give it time to "set."

Protect permed hair from the sun. Rinse out salt and chlorinated water immediately. Use as little heat from dryers or hot rollers as possible.

DRY HAIR: WHAT THE MODELS DO

Most models have dry hair, because it's been mercilessly manhandled. If yours is, too, stop doing so much to it. Maybe you're overdoing the shampoos, washing out the oils your hair needs to be smooth and shiny. Maybe you're applying too much heat too often, or you've overdone the chemical processing, or been burned by the sun. And, of course, it's just possible you are simply a dry-haired person. What to do?

- Wash (only one sudsing) *only* when your hair needs it. Use a mild shampoo designed for dry hair. Try plain castile shampoo.

- After exercise or a hot day, rinse the perspiration out and use conditioner. Perspiration is very drying.

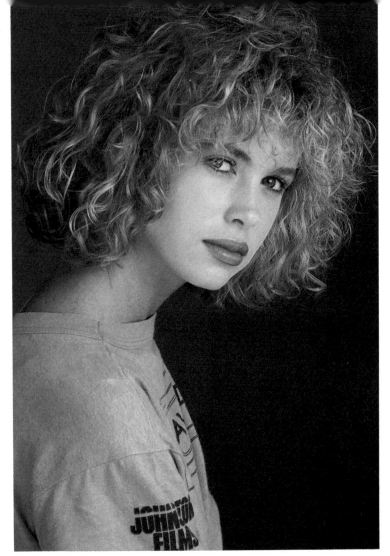

Hayley Mortison

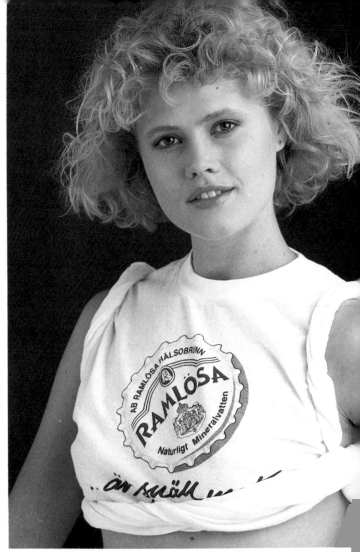

Eva Johansson

DRY HAIR is treated to a weekend emergency conditioning pack by Susan Hess. She applies the conditioner, ties her head up in a big scarf, and leaves it on as long as she can stand it.

• Dry your hair in the air whenever possible. Go easy with the heat. Use a medium or cool setting on your dryer, and just dry the roots. The ends will dry quickly on their own. Avoid direct sun and chlorine.

NO HAIR SPRAY, says Carrie Peterson. "It contains alcohol and it's drying." When she's on a job and in a hurry, she uses a natural plant gel to protect her hair from heat damage before using heated rollers or a dryer.

- Use a moisturizing conditioner every time you shampoo to coat your hair, seal in the moisture, smooth the hair and give it control.

- Give yourself a deep conditioning or an oil treatment every week.

SHARI BELAFONTE, *who's known for her Calvin Klein jeans commercials and can sing almost as well as her father, uses petroleum jelly for everything, including her hair when it gets dry. While her hair is still wet after a shampoo, she rubs just a little of it just over the surface of her very short Afro.*

- Trim off split ends frequently so the splits don't travel up the hair. Renée Simonsen, who's been on more magazine covers than I can count, has voluminous blond hair that's usually shoulder length. She makes sure her ends are trimmed about every four to six weeks. To minimize splits, she likes a very mild camomile shampoo.

FOR HER DRY HAIR, *Eva Voorhis doesn't shampoo every day. Instead she wets her hair and conditions it. After she brushes it out she then adds* more *conditioner to the ends. Furthermore, she declares she* never *uses heat on it. Neither does Jacki Adams unless a merciless hairdresser gets at her on a booking. Jacki washes her hair at night, lets it dry while she sleeps.*

OILY HAIR: WHAT THE MODELS DO

Hair needs oil to be healthy and shiny, but too much makes it limp, stringy and flat. The only solution is keeping it very clean, so plan to spend a lot of time under the faucet.

- Wash your hair every day, preferably in the morning, using a shampoo formulated for oily hair. Usually one sudsing is enough, but leave the suds on for a few minutes while you attend to the rest of you. Use warm water, not hot.

- Apply non-oily conditioner on the dry ends only.

- Keep your brush and comb scrupulously clean.

- Choose a simple hairstyle. With so much shampooing, you need a style that's easy.

- Set your hair dryer at medium or cool. High heat may activate sweat and oil glands.

- Final rinses: Give your oily hair a rinse with diluted lemon juice. *Or* dilute vinegar with water and pour it over your head last thing. *Or* blend two egg yolks with a couple of drops of lemon juice, leave it on your hair a few minutes before rinsing away.

- Don't wear tight hats or hair bands. Your scalp needs air.

- Comb, don't brush.

- Perms and coloring are well-known drying treatments for overly oily hair. They usually do a good job, at least for a while.

FINE HAIR: WHAT THE MODELS DO

Lots of models have fine hair, but they learn how to give it body and control. Their advice, and mine:

- Never use cream rinses.

- Don't shampoo more than necessary. Let some of the natural oils add body. On the other hand, too much oil drags hair down. Strike a balance.

- Use a light conditioner if it agrees with your hair. If it doesn't, don't.

- Think about a permanent. This can truly change your life.

- Think about coloring or highlighting to add body by roughing up the surface of the hair.

- Mousse, setting gels, sculpting lotions are *made* for you! Use your fingers as a brush, lifting at the roots as Julie Floyd recommends.

- Short hairstyles usually work best for fine, thin hair. Susan Hess says, "Gravity is the enemy. If the quality isn't terrific, the shorter the better." Eva Johansson wears her very fine, straight blond hair cut at chin length because it droops when it's longer.

VERY CURLY HAIR: WHAT THE MODELS DO

Though straight-haired women inevitably envy curly hair, those who have it often hate it. Is anyone ever happy? Try one or more of these tips gathered from our experts to tame very curly or frizzy hair:

- Don't wear your hair too long or too short. Medium length will give you better control.

- Mist with water and smooth down the ends when they curl up.

- Straighten it with soft jumbo foam rollers and a firm setting lotion, putting a fair amount of tension on the rollers.

- If it's coarse, use a cream rinse or cream-based conditioner and setting lotion.

- Don't brush if your hair is frizzy. Instead, use your fingers or a wide-tooth comb to lift and separate the strands.

- Don't wash it too much—mist it instead and/or add lotion for extra control.

- Check out reverse perming or "end smoothing"—it may relax the curl enough to please you as it does Shari Belafonte.

- Take advantage of mousse and gel to settle down frizzy hair. Work some through your damp hair with your fingers, stretching the hair with your head upside down.

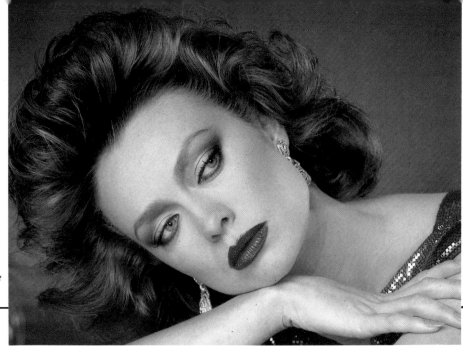

Vibeke

APRICOT OIL *is Susan Smith's solution to very coarse, very thick, very dry, sometimes frizzy red hair. She uses it as a hairdressing, putting a little on her palms and spreading it over her hair. It makes it manageable and adds the shine that coarse hair often lacks.*

- Use a moisturizing conditioner after *every* shampoo and a heavy-duty conditioner (or oil treatment) every week.

- For serious frizz, apply conditioner after the hair is *dry*. It will make it closer and flatter and shinier, too, says stylist Lois Pisani of the Pipino Buccheri Salon in New York.

- Spray a piece of cotton with hair spray; wipe upwards around your hairline to control the frizz.

- Add control with gels, sleeking your hair back and letting it dry that way.

EVA VOORHIS *uses pomade to help her thick, voluminous, curly hair stay in place. Ty Hendrick, on the other hand, prefers brilliantine to make her dark, wavy hair lie flatter to her head in the '40s look.*

- To unfrizz your hair, spray blow-dry lotion on damp hair. Take a section, roll it forward with a fat styling brush, and blow from the top to stretch the curl. The whole head done, brush down and then back.

- Have your very curly-frizzy hair cut in a great shape and enjoy it!

Anette Stai

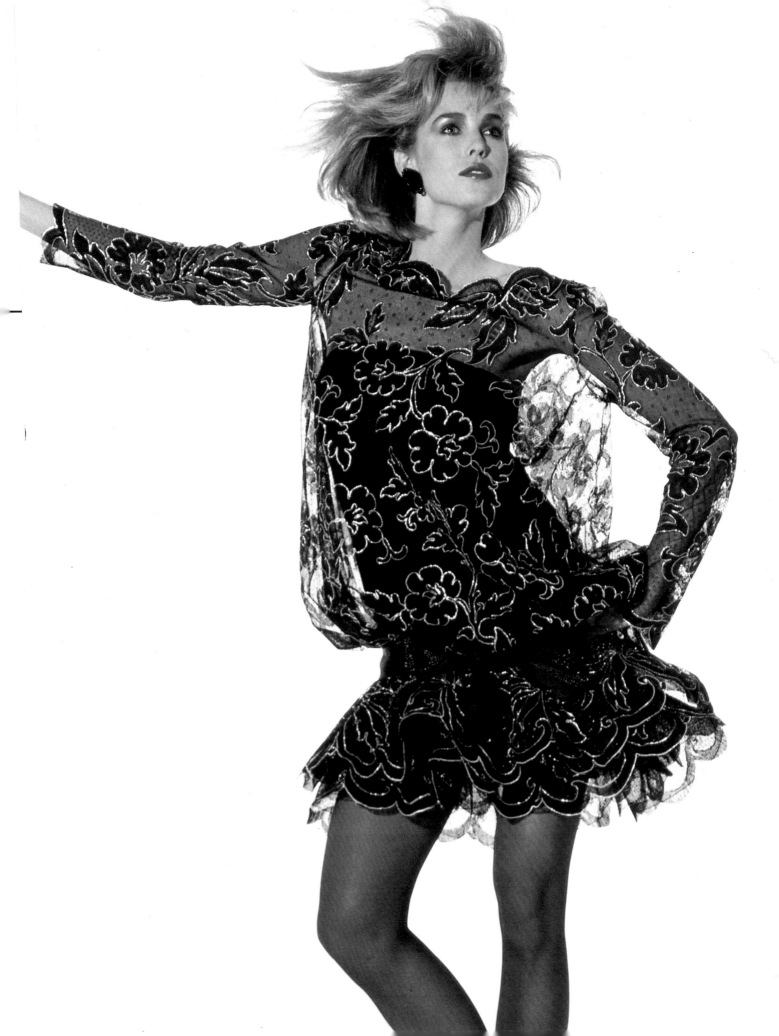

natural hair. Today it's used to accent, to brighten, to compliment your face, to make your own hair color come alive, not to change it into something unrecognizable. Even gray hair isn't turned into an imitation of what it once was, but simply tinted (or left alone) in a way that doesn't cry "Fake!"

The majority of Ford models who have color simply add highlights, while others lighten or darken only a shade or two. They use the color like makeup, a way to look better in a very natural way.

Even a subtle change can make a fantastic difference. When Debi Massey first joined us, we all agreed her mousey brown hair needed excitement. With subtle tone-on-tone coloring just a couple of shades lighter than her own, she became a dark blonde whose hair gleams and accentuates her big, blue eyes.

Maggie Fahy has her golden-brown hair highlighted right around her face about every two months. Carrie Miller adds highlights a shade or so lighter than her natural brown, and Rosie Vela's brown hair is given a warm golden glow that turns her into a dark blonde, enhancing an already exquisite face. Maura likes a few paler tones, too, near her face.

Except for adding some highlights, professional models rarely color their own hair. They don't *have* to because they are constantly attended by the world's best colorists. But home coloring today is so easy and so safe that you can experiment without danger of disaster. Leave permanent color changes to the specialists, and choose a temporary color that lasts one or two shampoos, or a semipermanent color that remains for perhaps six shampoos. Or add a mild bleaching product to produce subtle highlights, or lighten some strands here and there.

When you're doing the job yourself, says Louis Licari, color director of New York's La Coupe, be minimal. Don't try to make drastic changes. That's excellent advice because big changes require more knowledge and technique than any nonprofessional possesses. Licari is a big believer in no-peroxide colors "because you can't go wrong." If your hair turns out too dark to suit you, wash it, and it will lighten up. If it's too light, reapply the color to deepen it.

Remember that heat can strip color from your hair—use curling irons, blow dryers, hot rollers with caution, first applying a protective lotion. Cover your hair in the sun and wash chlorine and perspiration out immediately.

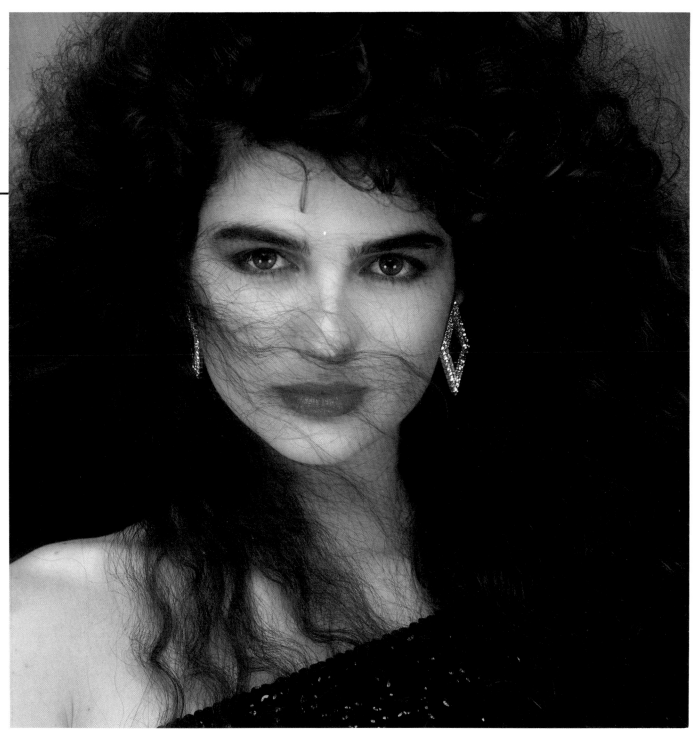

Eva Voorhis

HOME HIGHLIGHTS: HOW THE MODELS DO IT

Models spend more time in the company of hair stylists in one month than the rest of us do in a lifetime. No matter, many of them still prefer creating their own highlights on their own time. Usually they use commercial products, but sometimes they prefer to use kitchen colors like these.

FOR BLONDES AND LIGHT BROWNS

- Nancy DeWeir uses the old lemon-juice technique, combing the juice through wet hair before going out in the sun. Christie Brinkley recommends lemon juice, too, but likes to rub sesame oil into the ends to counteract the drying effect.

- Alda Balestra, whose shoulder-length hair is light brown, has an age-old European trick to suggest: Mix the lemon juice with camomile extract. White vinegar will also do a nice job of adding a glow, she says.

- Kim Charlton, the beautiful blonde who's married to our executive vice president, is a believer in camomile tea. She brews up a batch, lets it steep for 20 minutes, keeps it in a plastic jar in the refrigerator. After washing and conditioning her shiny blond hair, she pours some tea over her head and doesn't rinse it out. This mild treatment brings out soft highlights and acts as a light setting lotion, too.

- Donna Sexton sprays strong camomile on her blond hair when she goes out into the sun, says it gives subtle highlights to brown-haired friends, too.

- And Susan Hess mixes a little peroxide with sesame or sunflower oil, rubs it into her streaky blond hair, and goes out in the sun for an hour or so. The oil cuts the action of the peroxide, she says, giving nice natural highlights.

FOR BRUNETTES:

- Henna shampoo gives Laura Roberson's straight, thick, chestnut hair some lovely red highlights, especially in the summertime.

- Christie Brinkley's suggestion for brunettes is strong coffee or tea combed into the hair before sunning. Another way to accomplish the same wonderful highlights is mixing conditioner with strong espresso, applying it to clean, dry hair (damp if color-treated), covering with plastic wrap, and sitting under a dryer for ten minutes. This one comes from color expert Brad Johns.

- Neutral henna, of course, is the classic highlighter for dark hair. It's one several of our brown-haired models use to produce a sheen and a slight brightening.

- Or try these methods:

    —Mix dark rum with an egg yolk and add it to your shampoo.
    —Give your hair a cranberry-juice rinse for red overtones.
    —Combine camomile tea with red wine, use as a rinse to give brown hair a warm shine.

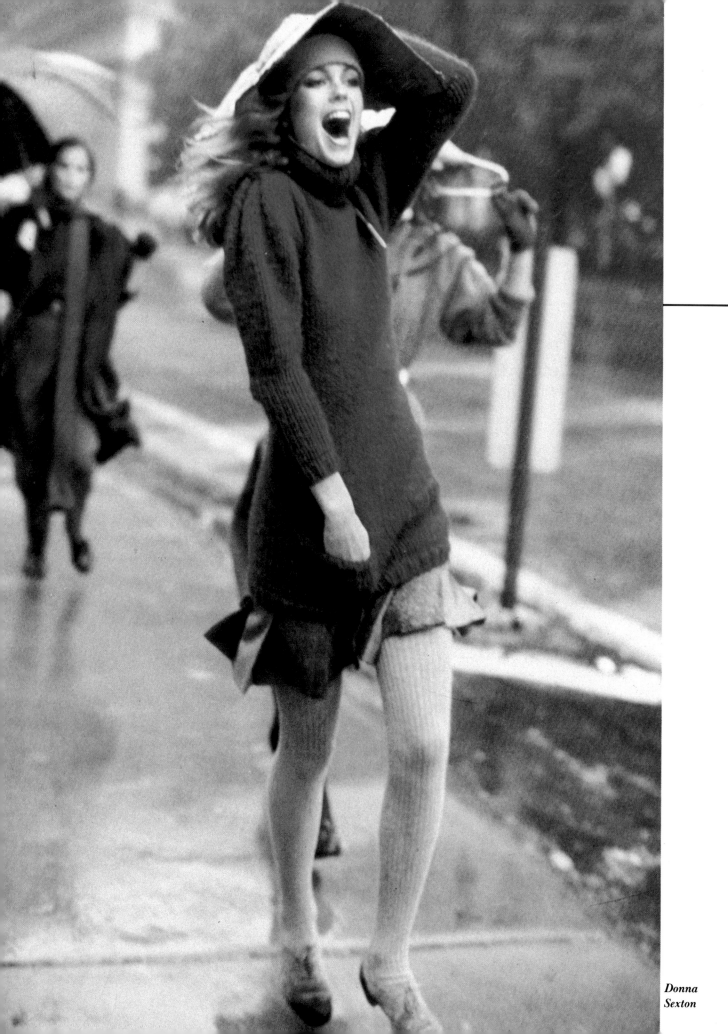

Donna Sexton

4

HOW TO HAVE MODEL HANDS

It may be hard to believe that models with their fabulous faces, their great smiles, their long lithe bodies, don't always have perfect hands and feet. But I'll tell you a secret—except for the hand models whose livelihoods depend exclusively on having the most beautiful extremities—often they're no better than yours or mine. Since they can't always hide them from the camera, models must learn how to make them look their best. And you should too.

Hands must always be meticulously groomed. Getting caught without a manicure is, to me, like getting caught without your clothes in the middle of Fifth Avenue. I learned the importance of groomed nails early. When I was about 25 years old and had just started becoming known as a model agent, I was invited to a party at *Vogue.* I went straight from the office in my scuffed suede shoes, my sweater and skirt, my chipped nail polish, and two nails that had broken off much shorter than the others. As I shook hands with the editor, an elegant man named Ira Patcevitch, he took that awful hand in his, looked at it, looked at me, and said in a soft sad voice, "My dear, even your toes should always be properly cared for."

From that day on, I've never gone out of the house without a manicure. Without a pedicure either, for that matter, because unattractive feet, though exposed less often, can be just as embarrassing.

Don't tell me you don't have time for manicures and pedicures. You do! Ford models are busy from early morning until late in the day, sometimes even into the night, often with only a half hour or so between bookings. They must learn how to give themselves a basic manicure and how to make emergency repairs. Though professional manicurists are usually in the studio when hands are an important element in a photograph and when the client has the budget for them, in most instances a model must fend for herself.

Most models simply keep their nails neatly manicured, without nail pol-

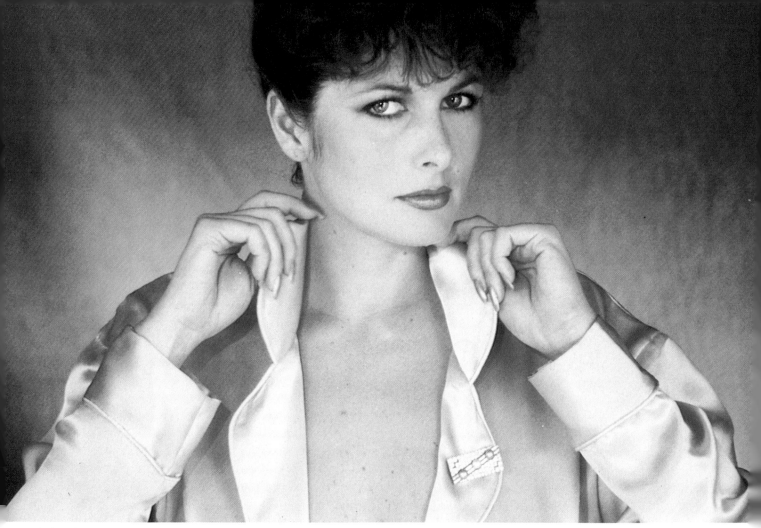

Cristina Ferrare

ish. If clients want them to arrive on the set with polish, that is specified when they book them.

Here's how we tell our models to care for their hands. Plus plenty of advice from our consultants and on-the-job hand-care tips from working models.

THE TRUTH ABOUT NAILS

Nails are dead, just like your hair, and there is no way you can change the way they grow except to protect them, camouflage them, and keep them from drying out. The purpose of nails is to protect your sensitive fingertips, help you pick up little objects, scratch your back, and maybe ward off danger.

Nails grow an average of an eighth of an inch a month, replace themselves in four to six months, and every single one of your 20 nails grows at its own unique rate, some noticeably faster than others on the very same hand. Your thumb is always the slowest. (Toenails grow much more slowly than fingernails.) You can't speed up the growth rate you've inherited, though one of our models swears she can make hers grow faster by continually tapping them lightly on a hard surface. I can't imagine tapping will do it, but it is certain to drive everyone around you crazy. It is definitely true, however, that nails grow faster in your teens, then slow up as you get older and may slow down abruptly when you're ill. They also grow more rapidly when you are pregnant and when the weather is steamy hot.

You can't improve your nails by swallowing gelatin. Simply eating a healthy, well-balanced diet with sufficient calcium and other minerals and nutrients is the most you can do for them, along with being careful not to abuse them.

If you mistreat your nails you can do real damage. They'll become dry and brittle, break off more readily, and look awful. Because nails are much more porous than the outer layer of your skin, overzealous use of polish, remover, nail hardeners, quick-drying preparations can take a toll, especially if you are not careful to replace oils and moisture. So will exposure to detergents, cleansers, and chemicals.

SKIN CARE FIRST

Obviously, rough red hands are unacceptable, model or not. And so are dry skin, ragged cuticles, bumps, lumps, and spots. The skin on your hands has fewer oil glands than your face and is constantly subjected to ill treatment, no matter how careful you are. So you must compensate for that. Every time you immerse your hands in water or you go out in cold or dry air, promptly apply lubricating cream.

Pat Tilley, whose hands were the stars of a well-known series of ads for Piaget watches and who has substituted her hands dozens of times in photographs for those of other more famous models, says, "When your hands feel dry, even if it's twelve times a day, cream them! I carry a little bottle of hand cream in my handbag so I have no excuses."

A good moisturizer helps, too, to ward off moisture loss. And always use sunscreen on your hands when you're out in the sun if you don't want to end up—a few years from now—with splotches and brown spots, along with wrinkles, all over the backs of your hands.

THE MODEL'S FRIEND: GLOVES

Every hand model in our agency—there are about 15 at any one time who specialize in hand shots—will carry on forever, if you let her, about rubber gloves!

Debra Secunda specializes in "spare parts" modeling and has been used in so many ads and commercials modeling her hands, neck and ears that, on one talk show, she was dubbed "The Queen of Parts." She is a rubber-gloves fan. "I always wear cotton-lined rubber gloves when I work around the house. Stuff a little cotton in the fingertips so your nails won't go through too quickly. That also takes the pressure off the tips of your nails when you're scrubbing pots." (Yes, models do scrub an occasional pot!)

Liz Attwood, who has been modeling both her hands and her feet for 18 years and obviously knows what she's talking about, keeps rubber gloves at every sink in her house. She also keeps a pair in her travel bag. By the way, the gloves slide on better if you dust a little powder inside them.

One of the best ways to keep your hands soft and smooth and to replace the oils you lose during the day is to wear cotton gloves to bed, if you can bear it. You should never go to bed without creaming your hands, but if they get the least bit chapped, do what model Jill Morris suggests: Smear your hands with petroleum jelly or a thick hand cream, pull on a pair of white cotton gloves, and go to sleep that way.

A MANICURE THAT LASTS

You need a manicure every week. The weekends are a good time for it, according to our busiest models because that sets you up for the work week. If your polish needs repairing before the week is up, learn to patch up the chips, as we'll explain shortly.

Most Ford models are quite expert at doing their own manicures. And if they're not, we send them to a manicurist such as Josephine Allen of Nails by Josephine Salon or Roseanne Singleton of Nails'n Things, both of whom specialize in elegant nails and are frequently hired on as part of the team on photographic shootings. There our girls learn how to cope with their own nails for the simple reason that they frequently don't have time between bookings to fit in a professional manicure when they need it. They learn all the basic techniques and emergency repairs as well.

Every model has discovered with horror, as she's rushed to a booking late and breathless, that she's broken a nail or chipped off some of her polish. She must know what to do in a hurry.

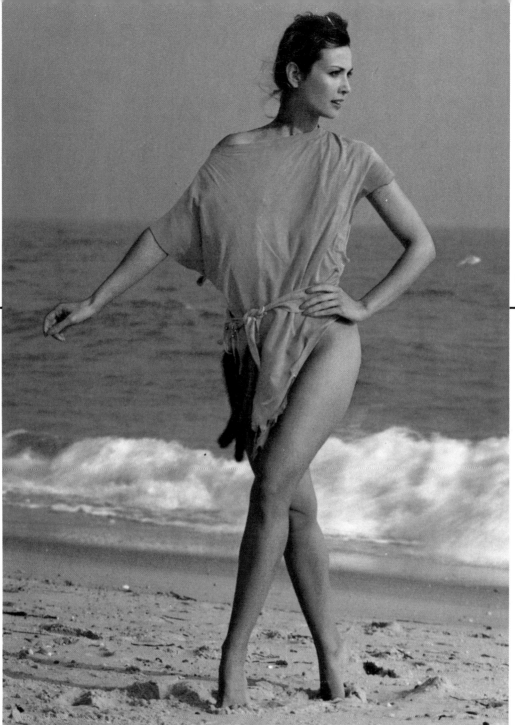

Debra Secunda

PRETEND YOUR POLISH IS WET, says hand model Debra Secunda. If you use your fingers as if you'd just given yourself a manicure, you'll save your nails. Do everything with the pads of your fingers, your knuckles, or something else like the eraser end of a pencil. Never use your nails as tools. If you must pick or scrape or push, find another instrument to do it with.

THE GREAT FORD MODELS' MANICURE

Here are the basic steps of a great home manicure, as outlined by Josephine, along with tips from Ford models.

STEP 1	STEP 2

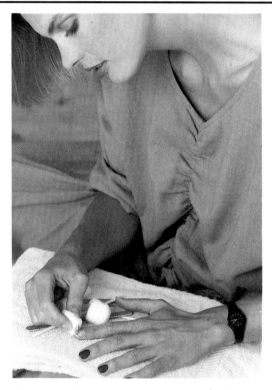

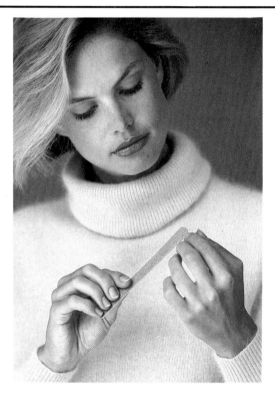

Using polish remover, take off your old polish. Soak a small piece of cotton in the remover and, starting at the base of the nail, wipe upwards to the tip until all polish is gone. To clean the remains of the stain off your cuticles, dip a cotton-tipped orange stick in remover and wipe around until you are pristine.

Shape your nails with an emery board, working on the underside of the nail and filing in one direction only, from the sides toward the center. Sawing back and forth tends to split the nails. (If your nails are very long, first cut off the excess with nail scissors or clippers *after* your bath when the nails are soft and pliable. If they're dry and hard, they'll split.) But they *must* be dry and hard before you file them. Never file wet nails, or they may peel.

Never file deep into the corners of your nails. This is the most common home manicuring mistake, and it sets you up for snags and splits and nails that snap off. Let them grow out straight and fairly square, then just round off the tips in a wide oval.

Model for pages 120–123: Sarah Stimson

**STEP
3**

**STEP
4**

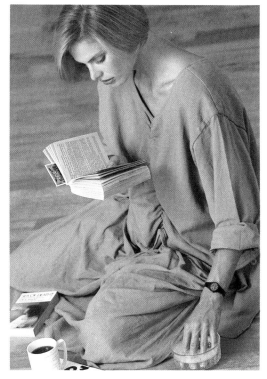

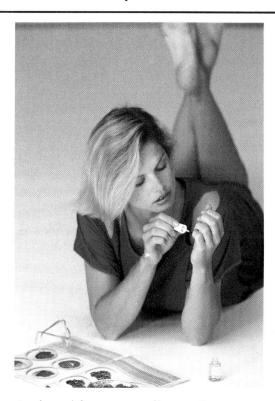

Add a few drops of oil to a small amount of body lotion. Heat it to lukewarm, then soak your fingertips for a couple of minutes to soften the cuticles and condition your nails. Wipe them dry. (If you skip this step in the interest of speed, then be certain to wash off all traces of remover with soap and water.)

Apply cuticle cream to all ten nails.

TAKE A BREATHER. *Give yourself a break occasionally and go a couple of days with totally bare nails except for cream. They can use a respite. Hand model Pat Tilley removes her polish every Friday night and leaves it off for the weekend.*

STEP
5

STEP
6

Carefully snip off hangnails with tiny manicure scissors, but do not cut the cuticles more than absolutely necessary or they will grow back thicker and heavier.

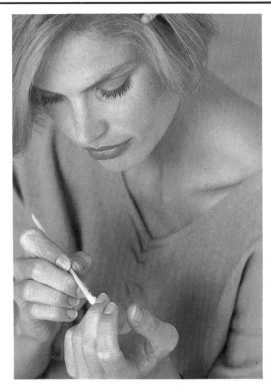

CUTICLE CARE. *To keep your cuticles supple, says Liz Attwood, massage cuticle cream into them every single day. It's heavier than hand cream, and Liz swears it makes her nails grow faster.*

IF YOU'VE SMUDGED A NAIL
while giving yourself a manicure and you're like me, you'll ruin more nails trying to fix it. Vanessa Angel, one of our English models, says to do repairs this way: Hold a little piece of remover-soaked cotton between the knuckles of your first two fingers of the other hand. Wipe the offending polish off that way, and you've saved your other fingers.

With an orangewood stick tipped with cotton, clean under your nails, and push your cuticles back very gently. Don't get too enthusiastic about this—your cuticles are there for a purpose. They protect the nailbed against injury and infection.

If it works better for you, use a special cuticle pusher or a Hindu stone to tidy up. A Hindu stone is like a little pumice stone which you dip into cream or water and use to push the cuticle back, smoothing the surface of the nail at the same time (great for toenails).

MAKE A MISTAKE? *Another tip from Debra Secunda, the "Spare Parts" model: Toothpicks are handier than orangewood sticks for cleanups. Used bare or with a bit of cotton wound around a tip, dip one into remover and gently remove misplaced polish. Or you can use a new gadget that looks like a pencil and comes with remover already in it.*

STEP 7

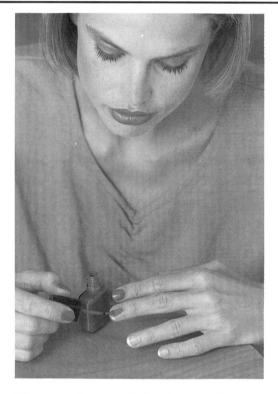

Rinse your hands and dry them, making sure to remove any oily residue from your nails or the polish won't stick. Apply a thin coat of base—too thick and it will bubble. Dip the brush into the base, wiping it off as you withdraw it. Make a stroke down the center of the nail, then on either side, from the base to the tip, covering the entire nail in these three strokes. Moons are out. Let it dry thoroughly, at least 5 minutes.

Now brush on two thin coats of nail polish, using the same three-stroke technique, allowing at least five minutes' drying time in between. Start all polish with the pinky of your dominant hand. You won't smear the finished polish so easily.

To minimize chipping, wipe a hairline of polish from the tip of the nails with your op-

STEP 8

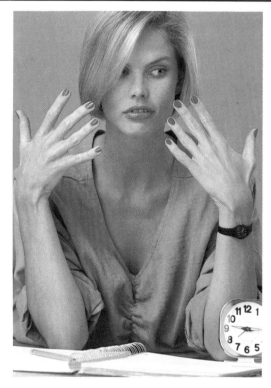

WAIT. Sit there with your fingers extended until the polish is truly dry, at least 20 minutes and preferably a lot longer.

Top coat or sealer is next. If your nails are brittle, you may want to use a nail hardener instead. Either way, be sure to "pull" it over the nail edges and dab some under the nails to prevent chipping.

WAIT. If you don't let your polish dry a good long time before bumping your nails against anything at all, you may have to start over again.

posite thumb while it's still wet. And, remember that the thicker the polish, the more likely it is to chip off like old paint. Keep the layers thin and smooth.

LIZ ATTWOOD, *a hand model who's kept so busy with bookings that she is always in a hurry, says: Don't dry polish with a hair dryer or under lights. You need at least an hour at a cool temperature for your polish to dry if you want to be really secure. Heat makes it bubble and shortens the life of your manicure.*

Quick-dry preparations don't really work, either, Liz states, because the polish underneath remains soft. Instead, try dipping your fingers in and out of ice water for a few minutes.

TIPS FROM THE TOP AND OTHER SOURCES

That's it for the basic manicure. Now here is a collection of helpful tips from both working models and our staff of consultants.

- *Buffing Your Nails.* If you don't want to be a slave to nail polish, try buffing. It's great for short and medium-length nails because it provides a good shine and improves the circulation of the nailbed. Long nails need nail polish!

  Here's how to buff: gently smooth out nail ridges, if you have them, with a fine emery board. This will also help remove yellow stain from constant use of polish or nicotine. Dab on buffing polish and buff your nails in one direction only, just long enough to produce a luster. Excessive buffing can thin the nails, making them subject to breakage, and once or twice a week is plenty often enough.

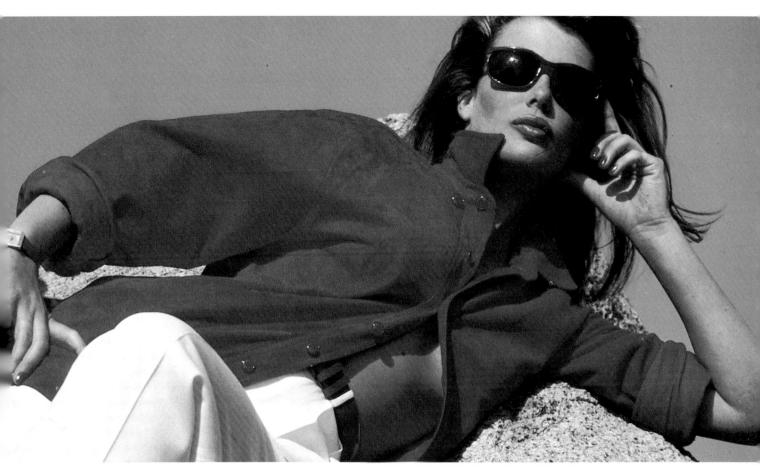

Kelly LeBrock

- *Coping With Ridges.* Gentle smoothing with a very fine emery board works for ordinary everyday vertical ridges. But if yours are really pronounced, maybe you'll want to use some ridge smoother or filler which will help smooth them out before adding a couple of coats of polish. Ridges are usually hereditary but sometimes are the result of iron or protein deficiencies (fad diet addicts, take note).

- *The Best Length:* Most women look best with medium-length nails that extend perhaps a quarter-inch beyond the fingertips. I've found that people with long, long nails become totally obsessed with them, worrying more about breaking one than crossing the street in front of a truck. I think there are more important things to think about. Besides, nails that look like claws are very unattractive. And they must be kept in perfect condition, neatly shaped, and *always* covered with polish.

CHERYL TIEGS, *one of our most famous Ford models, has more to say about long nails: "They obviously mean you're not doing anything very strenuous or life-enhancing like gardening or sailing. I think a good solution is a short, well-groomed nail, clean and glossy, coated with a clear polish which can be every bit as beautiful as a long red talon—and looks capable and natural."*

- *Not Too Stubby Either:* Very short nails—below the ends of the finger-tips—are not flattering to any variety of hand but especially if your fingers are not long and slim. One of our top fashion models, Debra Halley, says about her own hands: "I do not have good hands. They're too big, and my fingers are short—but nobody knows it. I keep them perfectly manicured and make sure my nails are quite long and polished. That gives the illusion of length. If your hands are not beautiful, they usually look best, too, with pale shades of polish. Bright red calls attention to them."

> **DEBRA SECUNDA:** *"Please be sure all your nails are the same length! It looks awful when you have one or two long nails and the rest are stubs—or vice versa."*

- *Make It Last:* To preserve your manicure for a full week, Josephine suggests a fresh coat of clear polish every other night. Pat Tilley always keeps a coat or two of the clear on her nails to protect the surface even when she doesn't wear polish.

BRITTLE NAILS: Here's what to do about them:
- Keep your nails from becoming dried out by protecting them with gloves in cold weather and wearing your rubber gloves for household chores. Use polish remover no more than once a week—it is a superdrying chemical. Be sure to wash it off when you do use it. Don't try to grow your nails very long—it won't work anyway, and you'll be kept busy repairing them. Keep them a moderate length and file them quite square. Over your polish, apply a coat of sealer every night, making sure you apply it under the tip too. Wear just the top coat to retard moisture loss if you don't like color.

- Nail hardeners can prolong the life of your polish and form a tough film over your nails, giving you some protection against breakage. Some even contain tiny nylon fibers for extra fortification. If you apply this stuff in a grid pattern, it is strongest. Maggie Fahy, whose nails tend to break, uses a base coat first, then a nail strengthener which she applies sideways across the nail first, then lengthwise.

- Once a week (or more if your nails are very brittle) soak your unpolished nails in warm water for 10 minutes, then dab on some oil or petroleum jelly to seal the moisture in. If you're on your way out, use moisturizer instead.

A HOT OIL TREATMENT *is what Debra Secunda gives her fingers for 15 minutes every week. Vitamin E oil is the magic ingredient for her, though others have told me they use olive or almond or even just plain baby oil. Remove your polish first so the oil can soak in. "The oil softens the cuticles," Debra says, "and it reconditions my nails besides."*

EMERGENCY REPAIRS

Even hand models, who treat their fingers like fine china, do break nails once in a while. Since their livelihoods depend on perfect nails, they fix them fast, and I'm going to tell you how they do it.

- *Chipped Polish.* This is an easy one. Don't remove all the polish from that nail. Simply do as Roseanne Singleton suggests: dab polish rather heavily on the vacant spot and let it dry completely. Then cover the whole nail with polish, smooth it all out with a layer of top coat, and you're almost as good as new.

- *Splits and Snags.* File down any rough edges immediately to prevent anything worse from happening. If your nail has split but it's still hang-

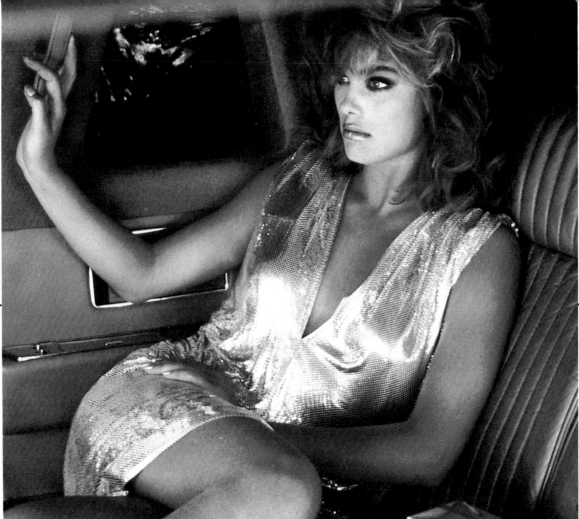

*Renée
Simonsen*

ing on, here's an easy fix from Josephine: Remove your polish and wash off the remover. Take a tea bag, open it, and empty out the tea. Tear off a small piece of the paper. Apply a dab of glue to the crack. Press a tiny bit of paper over it, then add some more glue. Let this dry thoroughly. With the fine side of an emery board, smooth the glued area. Cover with a layer of base coat and then polish as usual.

- *Broken Nails.* The easiest way to deal with a broken nail is to stick it back on again with glue and tea-bag paper in the same manner. Josephine tells the tale of going to Marlo Thomas's apartment in New York one evening to help her get ready for a gala movie premiere. Egad! Marlo had broken a nail! And she'd lost the piece! The intrepid manicurist cut off the tip of her own nail, shaped it, glued it onto Marlo's nail, and the day was saved.
Suppose you don't happen to have a spare piece of fingernail? Yours has broken off, and nobody offers you hers? You can buy little plastic nail tips in a kit and glue them on the same way, leaving them on until your own nails grow long enough.`

- *Nail Wrapping.* Models all know how to wrap their nails in an emergency, because there inevitably comes a time on location when there's no manicurist for hundreds of miles in any direction.
     Actually, the procedure is quite simple if you use a nail-wrap kit. You do require a little bit of nail to start with, which means you can't use this method if your nail has broken down very far. You must let it grow out far enough to have a small edge to work with.
Cut a wedge of the paper (substitute coffee-filter or tea-bag paper, if you like) to fit over your nail. Apply the adhesive to the paper, and stick it

onto your existing nail so that it extends about an eighth of an inch over the edge.

Smooth it out with an orangewood stick, and tuck the edges under the tip of your own nail. Now, with a little bit of remover on your opposite index finger, smooth it all out. Let it dry thoroughly, and then shape the tip with an emery board.

Now you're ready for base coat, two coats of polish, and a top coat.

NAIL BITERS' BULLETIN: *Aside from keeping your arms tied to your sides, the best way I know to stop this unattractive compulsion is to put on nail extensions. These are a liquid solution of acrylic, which hardens and sticks to your nails until they grow out. It's best to have them applied by a professional because they're tricky. They are not easy to bite.*

- *Nail Sculpturing:* If you simply can't grow your nails long enough to suit you, and you *must* have them, the way out is to acquire sculptured nails. This is not a do-it-yourself job for most of us. Frankly, I don't like the look of sculptured nails because they are rather thick and unnatural-looking, but some of our models love them. They do look great in a photograph, and they are truly tough and hard to break.

  It's done this way: A form is inserted under the nail, and the layers of a powder-oil mixture are built up until you have a nice long nail. The tricky part of this comes when your nails grow out after a week or two when you must have the grown-out area filled in and the ends trimmed.

- *Fake Nails:* I'm not even going to tell you how to apply those fake plastic nails that you glue on top of your own shabby set. You simply follow the directions on the package, sticking them on with special adhesive. I think they always *look* fake, and I've known several models who have had nasty allergic reactions to them. In an emergency, I suppose, they are useful. And, for nail biters, they are a good coverup that defies nibbling.

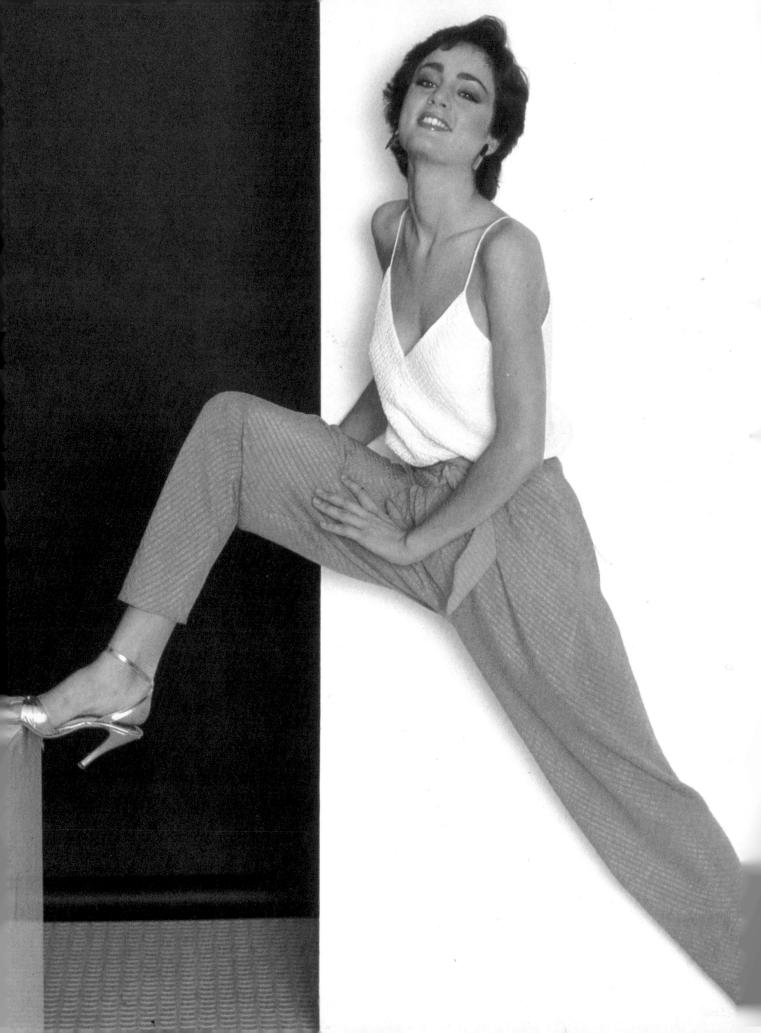

HOW TO HAVE MODEL FEET

Few of us think about our feet until they hurt. Models, however, *have* to think about theirs. For them, it's sheer economic necessity. On view all the time—a barefoot stroll down the runway wearing a swimsuit and nothing else, a shooting on location on a tropical island, posing in lingerie in a studio—their feet can't always be covered by shoes or tucked under a pile of sand. They must look good and it certainly helps if they feel good too.

ALL ABOUT FEET

Feet, each one of which contains 26 bones (a quarter of the body's total number of bones), 38 muscles, 56 ligaments, over 30 joints, are particularly susceptible to injury even though their soles are protected by skin 10 times thicker than the rest of the body. Toenails grow only a third to a half as fast as fingernails, and it may take them a year or more to replace themselves.

The average person takes 5,000 to 10,000 steps a day, and three out of four people stand on their feet more than four hours in 24. Models are on theirs more than that, often wearing shoes provided by stylists (who are more interested in trends than comfort) which don't fit and hurt besides. So we make sure they know, the minute they sign up with us, how to take care of their feet so they'll last a lifetime.

LOOKING GOOD

Let's start with foot care and tell you how Ford Models recommends keeping feet in good condition. It involves daily attention—you mustn't wait until your feet are in trouble, because by then a lot of damage has already been done and it may be irreparable. Every time you take a bath or a shower, for example, take the time to pumice off any hard, dry skin. When you get out, make a point of massaging them with body moisture and rub the nails with cuticle cream.

The following is the Ford plan for a weekly foot beauty and pedicure program. This is the basic routine. Variations come later.

STEP 1   Remove all nail polish.

STEP 2   Soak your feet. Fill a small tub with warm water and add a special foot-bath product or a little detergent or shampoo. Dip your feet in and stay there for 10 or 15 minutes. Now work on the callouses and rough stuff with a pumice or synthetic foot stone.

STEP 3   Dry feet thoroughly, making sure to dry between the toes. Remove traces of rough skin with one of those shaped foot files made for the purpose.

STEP 4   While your nails are still soft and supple, clip them straight across. Never, never cut them into the corners or round them off on the sides or you're likely to develop ingrown toenails. I've had them, and they hurt. Your nails should be no shorter than the ends of the toes and no longer than just a little beyond. Smooth with an emery board, filing in one direction.

STEP 5   Dab cuticle cream around the nails, massage it in, and push the cuticles back very gently with an orange stick, cuticle pusher or Hindu stone which smooths the nails at the same time.

STEP 6   Massage your feet and ankles with conditioning lotion.

STEP 7   Now you're ready for the finishing touches, buffing or polishing. Buffing is wonderful if you don't feel like maintaining perfect polish (see page 124 for directions).

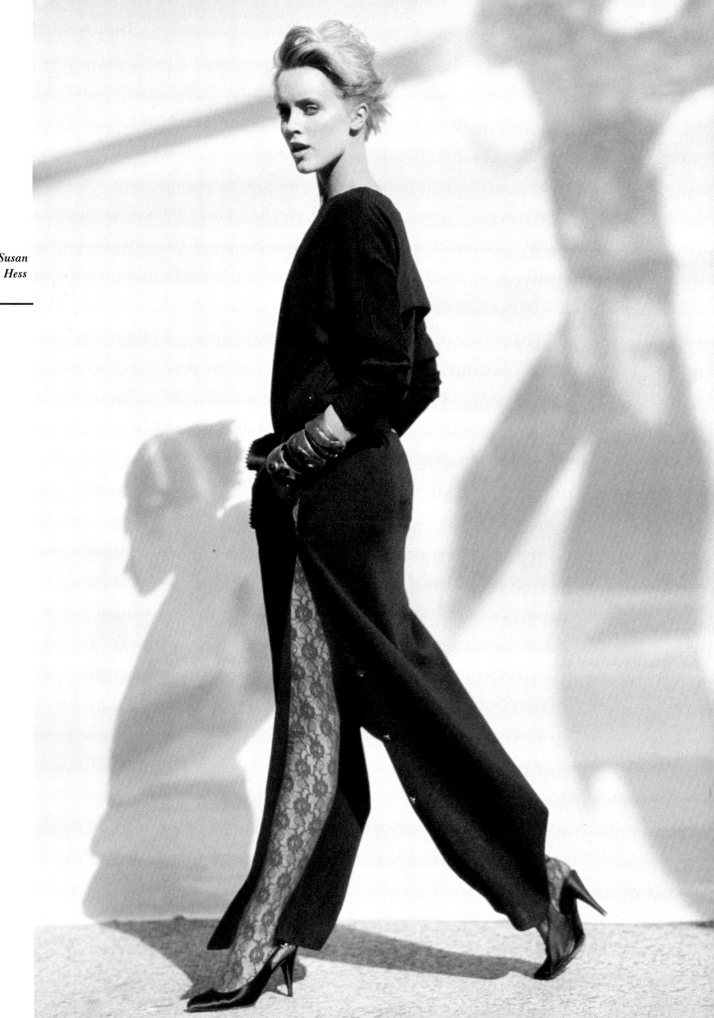

Susan Hess

If you've got vertical ridges on your toenails, buffing will help smooth them, though maybe you'll need to use the smooth side of an emery board.

If you're going to polish, first remove any residue of oil with polish remover and rinse it off. Make little wads of cotton or tissue and stuff them between your toes to keep them straight and separated. Give the nails a base coat, two coats of color, and a top coat (see the directions for a manicure, pages 120–23). If you don't want color, simply use a top coat.

Be sure to wait between each coat of polish long enough for it to dry thoroughly, or you'll be starting all over again. In a hurry, dip your toes in and out of icy water.

> **AN EXCELLENT WAY** *to be absolutely sure you've dried between your toes, thereby fending off athlete's foot, says foot model Lynn Thomas, is to use your hair dryer for a second or two. (But don't dry nail polish with heat.)*

FEELING GOOD

To keep feet comfortable and painless, you've got to practice preventive medicine. Ford models *never* wear high heels except on bookings or for a gala evening. In fact, most of them are seldom seen out of their running shoes (whether or not they are runners). I suggest doing as they do: carry a pair of running shoes or sneakers around with you. Wear them whenever you have to walk more than a block or two. I admit it looks weird to see a woman all dressed up and wearing a pair of those shoes on her feet, but it's such a common sight today that we can all get away with it. If you can't go that far, however, wear flats or low heels at least until you get where you're going and then change into higher heels.

CHERYL TIEGS, *who's written a couple of books herself, put it this way: "If you've already gone and bought a pair of unbelievably uncomfortable high heels . . . wear them for a couple of hours at a time only! The agonies of aching feet . . . will eventually show up graven on your face."*

All podiatrists agree that buying shoes that fit is the most important kind of preventive medicine you can practice. Never buy a pair that doesn't feel good right from the start.

ONE OF THE FORD MODELS *who runs around Central Park early in the morning, Willow Bay, the new Estée Lauder model, advises never stinting on running shoes. Buy good ones and make sure they fit perfectly. Don't wear the same socks twice; in fact, change your socks if they get too wet. Wash, cream, and moisturize your feet the minute you get back home.*

- Be sure your hose are big enough. It's just as bad to squeeze your toes with stockings as it is with shoes. Your toes should be flat out with or without stockings and not all pinched up.

- Wash your feet every day, dry and apply skin lotion. A few times a week, use a foot-buffing cream if you tend to get callouses.

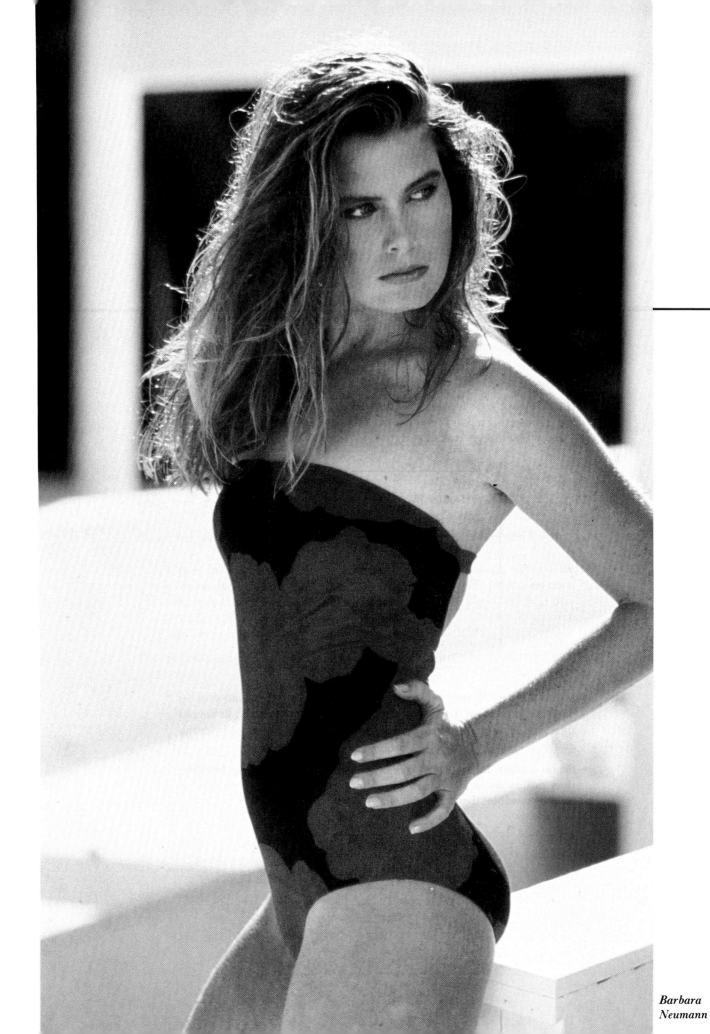

Barbara Neumann

6

THE FORD MODELS' QUICK SHAPE-UP DIET

Beauty is their business, so models watch their weight carefully. They can't afford the luxury of gaining too many pounds, because their bookings will drop off in a hurry. Clients resent paying $2,500 a day for a model who arrives at the studio too fat to fit into the clothes. That's bad for her business and it's bad for ours.

When a model needs to shed a quick five or ten pounds, we hand her the Ford Models' Quick Shape-up Diet. There are two versions and either one does the job. It takes off about a pound a day, so we don't advise staying on it for longer than two weeks at a time. Because it's very low in calories, yet quite nutritious, it's great for impatient people like me who don't like to wait for results. Although the Gourmet Cook's Diet does require some effort, the No-Cooking Diet is the easiest in the world.

When you reach the weight that's good for you, simply increase your portions and add some complex starches to your meals.

THE HEALTHY LOOK IS HERE

Models today are not superthin, though they have no flab or bulges. They look healthy and shapely, well-exercised and firm. The exceptions are the fashion-show models, especially those who work in Europe. They're what you'd call "skinny" because most designers insist upon it. At 5'9", for example, they may weigh as little as 110. That's fine if it's a requisite for making a living, but otherwise I don't recommend trying to be so thin. It is not attractive and it is not very healthy.

Occasionally, one of our models becomes too thin to photograph well and so we insist she put *on* some weight. But usually, like the rest of us, models have the opposite problem and that's when they receive a copy of our special diet.

THE FORD MODELS' DIETS: TWO CHOICES

There are many people who yearn to lose a few pounds and some who seriously embark on weight-loss plans. Some stick to them, others do not because, as a very overweight employee in our agency told me, "I don't like to cook." My instant reaction was, "Then stay fat." However, for once I curbed my sharp tongue and made a little survey. To my amazement, I found that at least 70 percent of our employees never cook at all! Some are addicted to fast foods or what I'd consider snacks. Others always eat out or buy prepared meals.

It's dismaying, but a fact of life today. I decided to find out how someone who never cooks can lose weight. I visited supermarkets and fish markets and other assorted food stores, and discovered how to do it. So I devised *two* diets: the Ford Models' Gourmet Cook's Diet for those who like to eat food prepared at home; and the Ford Models' Supermarket No-Cooking Diet for those who just won't or can't do it. Take your choice, or try one the first week and the other the second.

The Gourmet Cook's Diet is wonderful—it's so delicious that you won't mind being on a diet. The recipes are from my own collection or from our food-conscious models. Some are easy, others are more complicated, but they're all good. Follow this diet and you'll be amazed at how great you'll look in two weeks.

The Ford Models' Supermarket No-Cooking Diet is so simple you may laugh, but it will help you lose weight fast. Everything on the menus may be purchased at a supermarket, a prepared-foods shop, or a health-food store. Nothing requires more than heating up. Maybe two weeks on this diet will convince you you never want to cook again, or maybe it will have the opposite effect and you'll become a gourmet chef!

All the meals on both diets are interchangeable. Choose any breakfast, lunch or dinner, mix and match.

For beverages, drink whatever you want that has no calories, such as water, diet soda, seltzer, mineral water, tea, coffee.

Remember, stay on our low-calorie diet for no more than two weeks at a time. Check it out with your doctor before starting, as you should with any diet plan. With it, I suggest taking 1,000 units of vitamin C and one multi-vitamin daily.

Whatever diet you choose, you will lose the weight if you want to. Our models do, I do, and so can you.

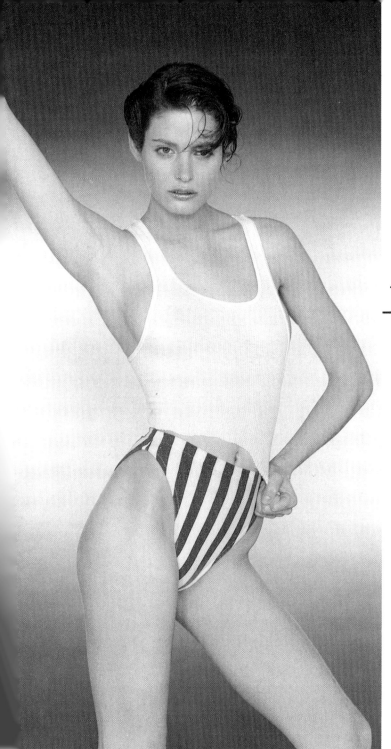

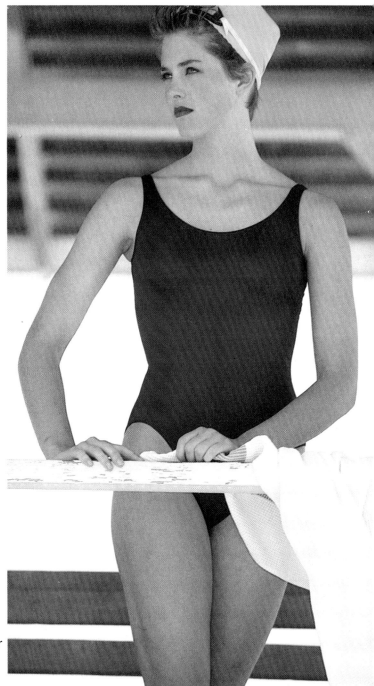

Jennifer Burry

Larisa Miller

THE FORD RULES

To be successful on a diet, any diet, you have to go by the rules. No cheating. Here are the most important rules and the ones I tell our models.

1. Cut back on your portions. Don't eat huge amounts of anything. In a restaurant, eat only half what's on your plate.

2. Skip the first course and the dessert—you don't need them. In our house, when we have guests, we serve dishes like asparagus or broccoli or spinach salad for a first course, and have fresh fruit for dessert.

3. Somebody once said, "Today is the first day of the rest of your life," and if you remember that, you won't let your life go by without achieving your goals. Start your diet now.

4. Never have any fattening foods in your vicinity. Get them out of your house. If they are not around, you can't eat them.

5. When you take your clothes off at night, take a look at yourself in the mirror. That should help motivate you!

6. Make being slender and healthy a part of your conscious being. It does not have to be your only topic of conversation, but keep it in your mind and think thin.

7. Make a habit of eating some celery, carrot or cucumber sticks about half an hour before dinner. Replace an alcoholic drink with vegetable juice or homemade bouillon. I make vegetable bouillon on weekends and freeze it in ice-cube trays. The homemade is great, but canned will certainly do in a pinch.

8. Drink a glass of water when you get up in the morning (I like it hot with a little lemon juice to cleanse the body), and two big glasses of water in midmorning and again in mid-afternoon. Drink another when you come home. This makes you feel full.

9. Don't boil vegetables, but steam them until they are just tender. They are more nutritious and delicious that way.

10. When you are traveling by plane, order your meals in advance. I always order a fresh fruit plate. If you can't do this, take along your own supply of fruit or raw vegetables.

11. Combine your dieting with the Ford Models' Quick Shape-up Exercise Plan. You'll lose weight faster and firm your body at the same time.

12. If the rest of your family doesn't need to lose weight, simply add rice or potatoes, beans or pasta to every meal for them.

WHAT THE MODELS DO (NO MATTER WHAT I SAY!)

Most of our models are sufficiently motivated by their desire to be superstars that they have no real weight problems. The vast majority don't need "a diet," but take action whenever they notice they've gained a little. That's the best way to do it. Here's how some models trim a pound or two off when necessary to stay in shape:

• *Renée Simonsen:* "When I gain a little, I eat only one kind of fruit for the whole day. For example, one day I eat only apples, the next only watermelon or pears. I can't eat too many because I get tired of them. Sometimes I drink only water for a whole day."

• *Willow Bay:* "I eat lots of foods with high water content, like lettuce, fruit, vegetables, and I drink lots of water. That fills me up."

• *Nancy DeWeir:* "I always have a problem with weight, more than other models do. If I didn't watch it, I'd be a blimp. I simply eat less of everything. Sometimes I fast for a weekend on nothing but juice and tea and vegetable broth. Or I go on Eileen's Supermarket No-Cooking Diet."

• *Ty Hendrick:* "I have a big bran muffin for breakfast, no butter, plus coffee and juice. Alcohol makes me gain weight, so I drink very little. If I'm dying of hunger, I eat plain popcorn."

• *Anette Stai:* "When I want to lose weight fast, I have boiled eggs, grapefruit and tea, three times a day. Plus as much cabbage as I can eat. And perhaps I add some dry Scandinavian crackers or whole-wheat bread. I always sit down and make a real meal of it."

• *Barbara Neumann:* "When I want to lose weight, I eliminate all alcohol and sugar and limit the dairy products. I fill up with sugar-free iced tea."

• *Alda:* "For a few days, I don't eat anything after 5 P.M. That gives my body time to burn the calories off and I don't go to bed loaded with food."

• *Anna Andersen:* "I exercise to lose weight. Or I go on a juice fast—fruit juice in the morning, and vegetable juice in the afternoon—for two or three days."

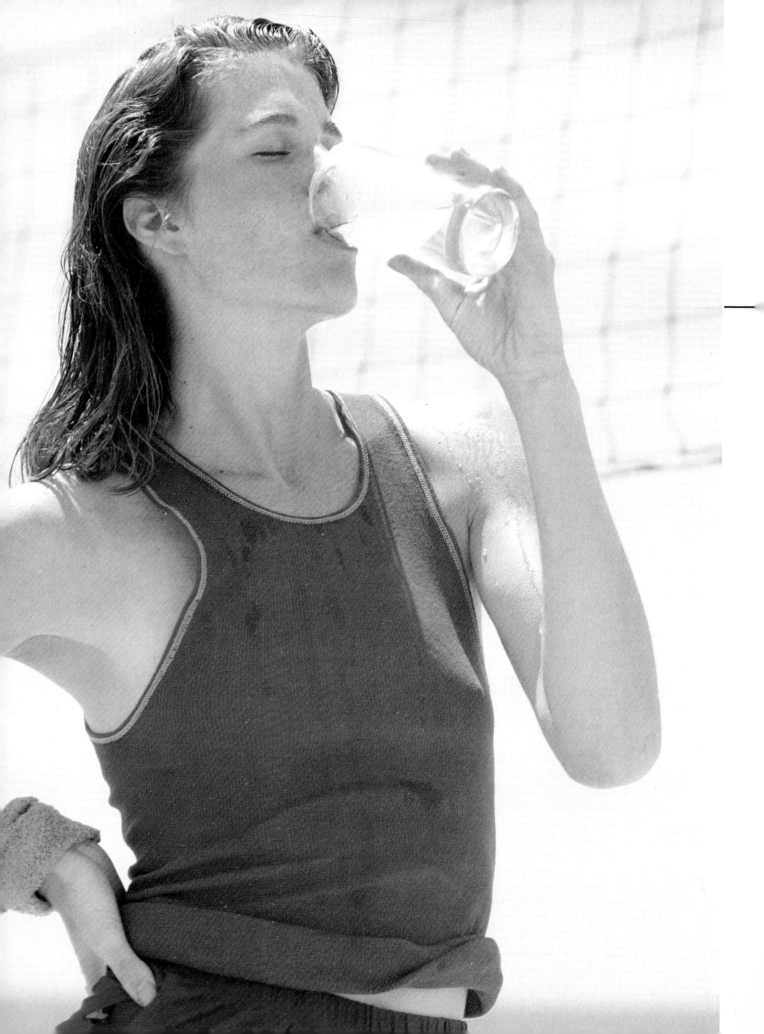

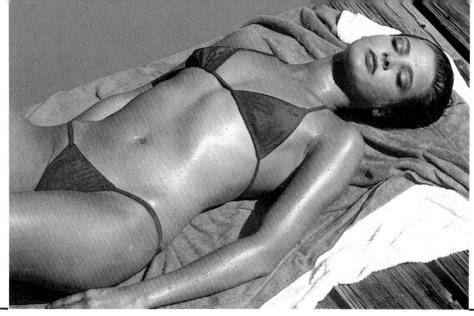

Donna Stia

• **Dianne deWitt:** "I'm always trying to *gain* weight. All those runway shows and the traveling make me get too thin. I just eat more. I especially like vegetables and fish and I never eat red meat."

• **Jennifer Berrington:** "I was one of those models who ate myself out of business for a while. I cut back on *everything* and drank lots of water."

• **Donna Stia:** "I have to think about my weight every day of my life. I do a lot of walking and jogging, and I make sure my portions are very small and low in fats. To lose in a hurry, I go on a very low-calorie diet like the Ford Models Diet."

• **Micaela Sundholm:** "I get too thin very easily, and I have to keep eating constantly. I try to eat high-calorie, high-nutrition foods like milk products and cranberry juice."

• **Carrie Peterson:** "I love to eat and I have to be careful. If I have a heavy meal, the next day or two I just eat fruit for breakfast and vegetables for lunch and have a balanced dinner. Salad has very little value, so I try to eat vegetables like broccoli and carrots, always undercooked."

• **Rosemary McGrotha:** "For a while, I was too fat for a model. I tried every diet and finally I went on the Ford Models Diet which worked."

• **Vibeke:** "If I gain a few pounds, I stop eating completely. It's no fun, but there are no miracles and you have to give up certain things in life. I just have water, soup, juice, tea and coffee. For me, it's everything or nothing."

• **Shari Belafonte:** "If I eat fruit or vegetables before my meal, it keeps me from overeating."

Now, here are our two Ford Models diets. We'll start with the no-cooking diet because nothing could be easier. Though a few of our models love to cook and so prefer the gourmet cook's diet, most of them want to be minimally involved with food preparation.

Remember you can choose any breakfast, lunch or dinner, mixing them each day as you like.

*Martha
Longley*

THE FORD MODELS' NO-COOKING SUPERMARKET DIET

A TWO-WEEK PLAN

DAY

1

BREAKFAST

½ medium grapefruit (if you have a serrated grapefruit spoon, all you have to do is remove the seeds)
1   cup puffed wheat
1   cup skim milk
4   strawberries

DAY

2

BREAKFAST

1   cup strawberries
    or
½ medium grapefruit
1   slice gluten bread, toasted with
1   teaspoon low-calorie margarine
1   cup skim milk

DAY

3

BREAKFAST

½ cantaloupe
5   rye Melba toast
1   hard-boiled egg
1   cup skim milk

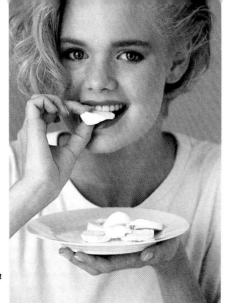

Anna Magnusson

LUNCH

1 cup garden low-fat cottage cheese, with some watercress, lettuce, etc., from produce department or salad bar
1 slice whole wheat bread

DINNER

1 cup beef bouillon made from a cube
4 ounces waterpacked tuna (add dried dill, a bit of tabasco and mix in a little onion powder)
Salad of mixed greens
1 tablespoon low-calorie dressing
1 large apple

LUNCH

From salad bar in supermarket, mix lots of vegetables with lettuce and
1 tablespoon low-calorie dressing
1 slice whole wheat bread
1 apple

DINNER

1 portion frozen Moo Goo Gai Pan (or ½ portion from Chinese take-out)
1½ cups heated stewed tomatoes

LUNCH

1 cup low-fat cottage cheese with chives and green pepper wedges
3 long thin bread sticks
1 banana

DINNER

1 cup tomato juice
¼ barbecued chicken from supermarket or takeout. Eat white meat only, no skin
Cucumber salad from salad bar

DAY
4

BREAKFAST

½ grapefruit
1 cup puffed rice with 4 strawberries
1 cup skim milk

DAY
5

BREAKFAST

1 slice pineapple ¾″ thick, 3″ across
   (can be cut at market)
1 cup puffed wheat
1 cup skim milk

DAY
6

BREAKFAST

½ medium grapefruit
1 hard-boiled egg
1 cup skim milk

LUNCH

1   shrimp cocktail in a jar
½   peeled cucumber
⅛   small tomato with a light sprinkle of salt
1   slice whole wheat bread
1   teaspoon margarine

DINNER

1   frozen turkey dinner
Green salad with
1   tablespoon low-calorie dressing
1   slice watermelon

LUNCH

1   cup mixed fresh fruit
1   cup yogurt
    Salad from salad bar—low-calorie dressing
10 Melba rounds

DINNER

1   cup tomato juice, hot or cold
4   ounces cooked lobster (can be canned)
1   tablespoon low-calorie mayonnaise mixed with dried tarragon
1   cup spinach salad with 1 tablespoon low-calorie dressing

LUNCH

2   frozen shrimp egg rolls (meatless)
Sliced tomatoes
Carrot
Cucumber
Celery sticks

DINNER

1   cup V-8 juice, hot or cold
4   ounces cooked Alaskan king crab-meat
1   teaspoon low-calorie mayonnaise
1   cup spinach salad with
1   tablespoon low-calorie dressing
½   cantaloupe

DAY

7

BREAKFAST

½   cantaloupe
1   deviled egg (mix yolk of hard-boiled egg with 1 teaspoon Durkee's Famous Dressing)
1   cup skim milk

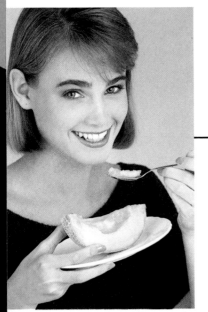

Joyce Hartenstein

DAY

8

BREAKFAST

½   medium grapefruit
1   cup puffed rice
½   small banana
1   cup skim milk

DAY

9

BREAKFAST

½   cantaloupe
4   pieces Finn Crisp
1   cup skim milk

LUNCH

2 cups fruit salad with yogurt and dried mint

DINNER

1 cup tomatoes, cucumber and mushroom salad. Sprinkle with dried or fresh dill

4 ounces cooked breast of turkey or chicken (no skin)

1 cup vegetable salad (no sprouts or chick peas) with

1 tablespoon low-calorie dressing

LUNCH

3 ounces water-packed tuna with lettuce, any fresh herbs you can find

1 tablespoon low-calorie dressing

1 slice whole wheat bread

1 apple

DINNER

4 ounces of kielbasa and sauerkraut (buy it already cooked at the supermarket). Heat and eat with a tiny bit of mustard as a dip. You can add more sauerkraut but not sausage.

Raw spinach salad with sliced mushrooms and low-calorie dressing

LUNCH

4 ounces fresh fruit salad. Buy premixed or cut up cantaloupe, honeydew, grapefruit sections and strawberries (no bananas).

½ cup cottage cheese

DINNER

1 frozen Cantonese chicken dinner

Large lettuce salad

1 tablespoon low-calorie dressing

DAY
10

BREAKFAST

½ medium grapefruit
1 cup puffed wheat
6 strawberries
1 cup skim milk

DAY
11

BREAKFAST

1 medium eating orange
1 small toasted pita bread
1 teaspoon low-calorie margarine
1 cup skim milk

DAY
12

BREAKFAST

½ medium grapefruit
1 small pita, toasted
1 teaspoon low-calorie margarine
6 dried prunes
1 cup skim milk

LUNCH

1 cup low-calorie cranberry juice
2 Finn Crisps spread with
1 teaspoon low-calorie cheese spread (If you spread it very thin, have 3.)
1 hard-boiled egg
4 ounces cucumber salad from salad bar (If you feel energetic, add a sliced radish.)

DINNER

4 ounces prepared cooked haddock from deli department
Raw vegetable salad with broccoli, cauliflower, 2 cut-up scallions, 1 cut-up carrot. Try my oilless salad dressing to which you can add 1 tablespoon grated Romano cheesc
¼ honeydew melon

LUNCH

½ cantaloupe filled with
½ cup low-fat cottage cheese
10 Melba rounds
Lettuce salad
1 tablespoon low-calorie dressing

DINNER

1 can steamed clams with broth, heated
1 small ear boiled corn or ½ cup canned corn kernels
1 teaspoon low-calorie margarine
Large lettuce salad
1 tablespoon low-calorie dressing

LUNCH

2 cans asparagus, drained
2 ounces low-fat mozzarella
4 ounces cucumber, onion and tomato salad from salad bar
1 tablespoon low-calorie dressing

DINNER

8 ounces frozen Alaska king crab, defrosted and drained
Raw spinach and mushroom salad with 1 teaspoon grated Romano cheese
½ cantaloupe or 1 small orange

Sarah Stimson

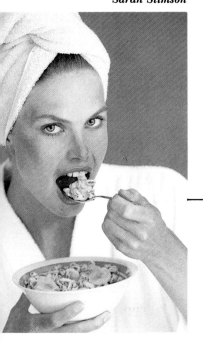

DAY
13

BREAKFAST

1   slice pineapple, ¾″ thick by 3″ across
½   toasted English muffin
1   teaspoon low-calorie margarine
1   cup skim milk

BREAKFAST

1   small orange
1   slice whole wheat bread, toasted
1   teaspoon low-calorie margarine
1   cup skim milk

DAY
14

(The menu for this day is designed to be eaten on a Sunday, when many people eat their main meal at midday. You can easily reverse the sequence of these two meals as I've indicated.)

LUNCH

2 canned artichoke bottoms (don't buy artichokes in oil—these are usually French and should be washed before eating). Top artichokes with
3 ounces canned crab meat mixed with 1 teaspoon chives and 1 tablespoon low-calorie dressing
1 apple
1 cup V-8 juice, heated

DINNER

3 ounces lean roast beef
1 cup frozen cooked Brussels sprouts or broccoli
Lettuce salad with cucumber, green pepper and perhaps some spinach
1 teaspoon oilless dressing

LUNCH (or SUPPER)

Tuna melt made of 2 ounces water-packed tuna, well drained and mixed with a little chopped onion, dried dill and a few drops of Tabasco (optional). Place on top of 2 Finn Crisps. Cover with 1 ounce low-fat mozzarella and put in oven until cheese is melted.
Carrot, cucumber and celery sticks—as much as you wish.

SUPPER (or LUNCH)

½ can Petite Marmite soup, heated
1 frozen Chinese shrimp puff, heated in oven
4 ounces white meat turkey (no skin)
3½ ounces frozen spinach, cooked
Raw vegetable salad, mixed with
1 tablespoon low-calorie dressing to which you may add
½ teaspoon finely chopped garlic and
1 teaspoon low-calorie yogurt

THE FORD MODELS' GOURMET COOK'S DIET

A TWO-WEEK PLAN

DAY 1

BREAKFAST

½ medium grapefruit
1 cup puffed wheat
1 cup skim milk
4 strawberries

DAY 2

BREAKFAST

1 cup strawberries
1 slice cracked wheat bread
1 teaspoon low-calorie margarine
1 cup skim milk

DAY 3

BREAKFAST

¼ cantaloupe
5 rye Melba toasts
1 teaspoon margarine
1 ounce mozzarella cheese
1 cup skim milk

* Recipes for foods followed by an asterisk appear immediately following this menu section.

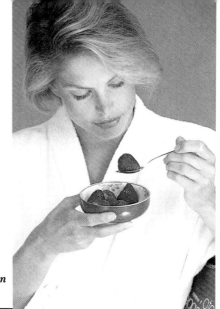

Sarah Stimson

LUNCH

1 slice whole wheat bread
1 teaspoon low-calorie margarine
1 cup watercress salad with oilless dressing*

DINNER

1 cup mushroom bouillon (cold or hot)*
1 slice Sicilian broiled swordfish*
1 cup steamed broccoli
2 cups green salad with tarragon dressing

LUNCH

1 cup spinach mold* with tomato coriander sauce*
1 small banana

DINNER

1 fillet blackened fish*
1 cup steamed spaghetti squash or zucchini
1 cup orange cabbage*
Lettuce salad with oilless dressing*

LUNCH

1 cup low-fat cottage cheese mixed with chopped green pepper, diced cucumber, radish and chives
1 small pita
1 navel orange

DINNER

2 steamed chicken sandwiches*
1 cup stir-fried spinach*
Watercress salad with oilless* or any low-calorie dressing

DAY

4

BREAKFAST

½ medium grapefruit
1   cup puffed rice with
1   cup skim milk

DAY

5

BREAKFAST

1   medium eating orange
1   egg, scrambled in nonstick pan
½ toasted English muffin
1   teaspoon margarine
1   cup skim milk

DAY

6

BREAKFAST

1   medium grapefruit
1   boiled or poached egg
5   slices Melba toast
1   cup skim milk

LUNCH

Lots of spinach and mushroom salad with low-calorie dressing
½ whole wheat English muffin
1   teaspoon margarine
1   apple

DINNER

1   cup Trini salad*
4   ounces salt chicken,* white meat only
1   cup steamed broccoli with lemon

LUNCH

Lots of carrots, watercress, celery and cherry tomatoes
1   cup low-fat cottage cheese
10 Melba rounds

DINNER

1   cup tomato bouillon*
6   ounces herb-broiled halibut*
1   cup spinach with onion powder*
¾   cup steamed carrots

LUNCH

2   medium cans of asparagus tips
1   cup cold steamed broccoli with lemon juice
2   large bread sticks
1   small piece of fruit

DINNER

Raw vegetable salad*
8   garlic baked shrimp*
1   cup steamed Brussels sprouts

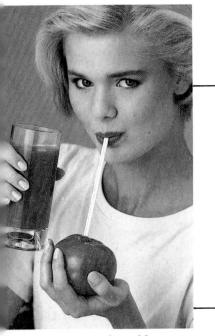

Anna Magnusson

DAY 7

BREAKFAST

½ medium grapefruit
1   frittata (1 egg mixed with 1 table-
    spoon each: chopped green peppers,
    scallions and low-fat yogurt plus 1
    chopped mushroom, fried in non-
    stick pan. Do not stir.)
1   cup skim milk

DAY 8

BREAKFAST

½ medium grapefruit
1   cup puffed rice
1   cup skim milk
½ banana

DAY 9

BREAKFAST

½ cantaloupe
4   pieces Finn Crisp
1   cup skim milk

LUNCH

Crudités*
4 ounces bass in foil*
Herb grilled tomato salad*
1 banana or orange

DINNER

1 cup chicken salad
1 crisped potato skin with low-fat ricotta cheese and low-fat chives dip
1 cup steamed broccoli

LUNCH

3 ounces water-packed tuna, mixed
  with chopped onion and powdered
  dill
½ English muffin
1 medium can asparagus or 10 fresh
  steamed asparagus
1 cup berries

DINNER

Warm mushroom salad*
4 ounces peppered swordfish steaks*
½ cup steamed broccoli with lemon
  juice
Lettuce salad with oilless salad dressing*

LUNCH

12 boiled shrimps
1 teaspoon cocktail sauce
1 bunch celery with outside stalks removed
1 small roll
1 teaspoon margarine
1 navel orange

DINNER

1 cup tomato juice
4 ounces poached bass*
1 cup steamed spinach
Watercress and grapefruit-section salad
with oilless dressing*

DAY
10

BREAKFAST

½   medium grapefruit
1   cup puffed wheat
1   cup skim milk
6   strawberries

DAY
11

BREAKFAST

1   medium eating orange
1   small toasted pita bread
1   teaspoon low-calorie margarine
1   cup skim milk

DAY
12

BREAKFAST

½   medium grapefruit
8   dried prunes
1   poached egg
1   slice whole wheat bread
1   cup skim milk

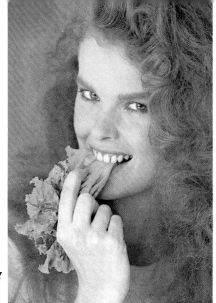

Kathryn Redding

LUNCH

3 slices white meat turkey
4 slices tomato with basil
1 slice whole wheat bread
1 teaspoon low-calorie margarine or mayonnaise
1 apple

DINNER

1 cup low-calorie cranberry juice
6 ounces Chinese chicken*
1 cup steamed broccoli with lemon
Raw spinach salad with low-calorie herb dressing

LUNCH

½ cantaloupe filled with ½ cup low-fat cottage cheese
10 Melba rounds
Lettuce salad with low-calorie dressing

DINNER

2 broiled lamb chops, fat removed
4 ounces watercress purée*
1 grilled tomato
1 fresh pear

LUNCH

1 cup beef bouillon
Raw vegetable salad with broccoli, cauliflower, shredded cabbage, chopped fennel
1 tablespoon low-calorie dressing or 2 tablespoons oilless dressing*
1 toasted English muffin
1–2 teaspoons low-calorie margarine

DINNER

4 ounces baked salmon*
Large mixed salad with lettuce, cucumber, scallions, cherry tomatoes
Oilless dressing*
½ cantaloupe

DAY
13

BREAKFAST

1   slice pineapple, ¾″ thick, 3″ across
½   toasted English muffin
1   pat low-calorie margarine
1   cup skim milk

DAY
14

BREAKFAST

½   medium grapefruit
1   egg scrambled in top of double boiler
    with 1 tablespoon diet margarine
1   slice toasted gluten bread
1   teaspoon low-calorie margarine
1   cup skim milk

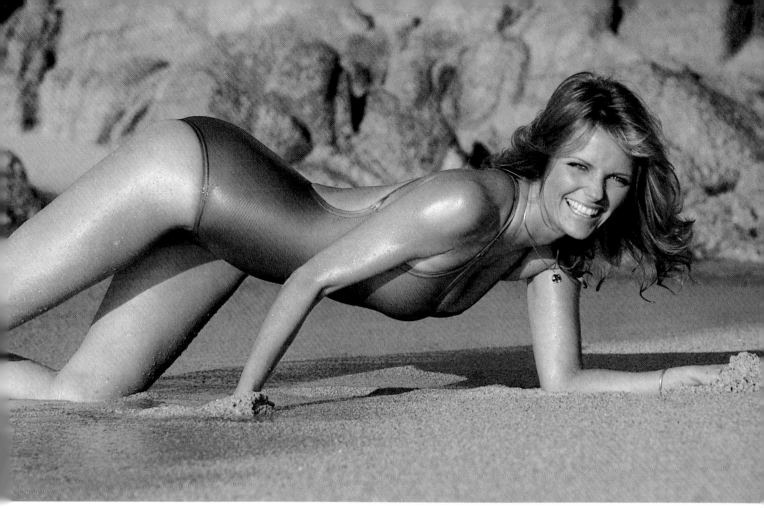

Cheryl Tiegs

LUNCH

Hot vegetable juice
Fruit salad made with cantaloupe, apple, grapefruit, orange
1   tablespoon low-calorie mayonnaise, on lettuce
4   Finn Crisps

DINNER

1   cup herbed tomato soup*
1   cup sautéed scallops*
1   cup puréed spinach*
Chopped lettuce salad
Herb dressing
¼   honeydew melon

LUNCH (or SUPPER)

1   cup beef or chicken bouillon
Chef's salad made with
1   ounce white meat turkey
1   ounce Parmesan cheese in small pieces
1   ounce lean ham
4   cherry tomatoes
Lots of lettuce
Low-calorie dressing
1   toasted pita bread
1   teaspoon low-calorie margarine

SUPPER (or LUNCH)

4   ounces herb roasted chicken*
1   cup zucchini mold with tomato sauce*
Large lettuce salad
Low-calorie dressing
1   pear or peach

FORD MODELS' GOURMET COOK'S DIET RECIPES

MUSHROOM BOUILLON   (Day 1 Dinner)

3   stalks of celery
1   onion
1   carrot
3   cups water
1   quart chicken bouillon
1   pound (2 cups) finely chopped mushrooms
Salt (optional)

Chop celery, onion and carrot. Simmer in 3 cups of water for 45 minutes. Strain and add chicken bouillon. Add the chopped mushrooms and perhaps a little salt. Cook for five more minutes and serve hot or cold.

SICILIAN BROILED SWORDFISH (Day 1 Dinner)

1   thin slice (4 ounces) swordfish steak per person
1   teaspoon olive oil per steak
Rosemary
Salt (optional)

Brush each steak with a little oil and coat heavily with rosemary and a light sprinkle of salt if you wish. Preheat broiler. Place swordfish steak on broiling pan and broil about 4 inches from the flame. Baste fish occasionally with oil until cooked (about 15 to 20 minutes). Don't turn. Serve at once.

SPINACH MOLD (Day 2 Lunch)

1   cup frozen chopped spinach, thawed and drained, per serving
2   tablespoons low-fat ricotta cheese per serving
1   pinch nutmeg per serving
2   egg whites, beaten until stiff per serving

Combine spinach, ricotta and nutmeg in a bowl. Carefully fold egg whites into mixture and spoon into custard cups. Place cups in a pan of water that reaches almost to the top of the cups and bake in preheated 350° F. oven until firm (about 25 minutes). Serve at once with tomato coriander sauce or plain.

Patricia Van Ryckeghem

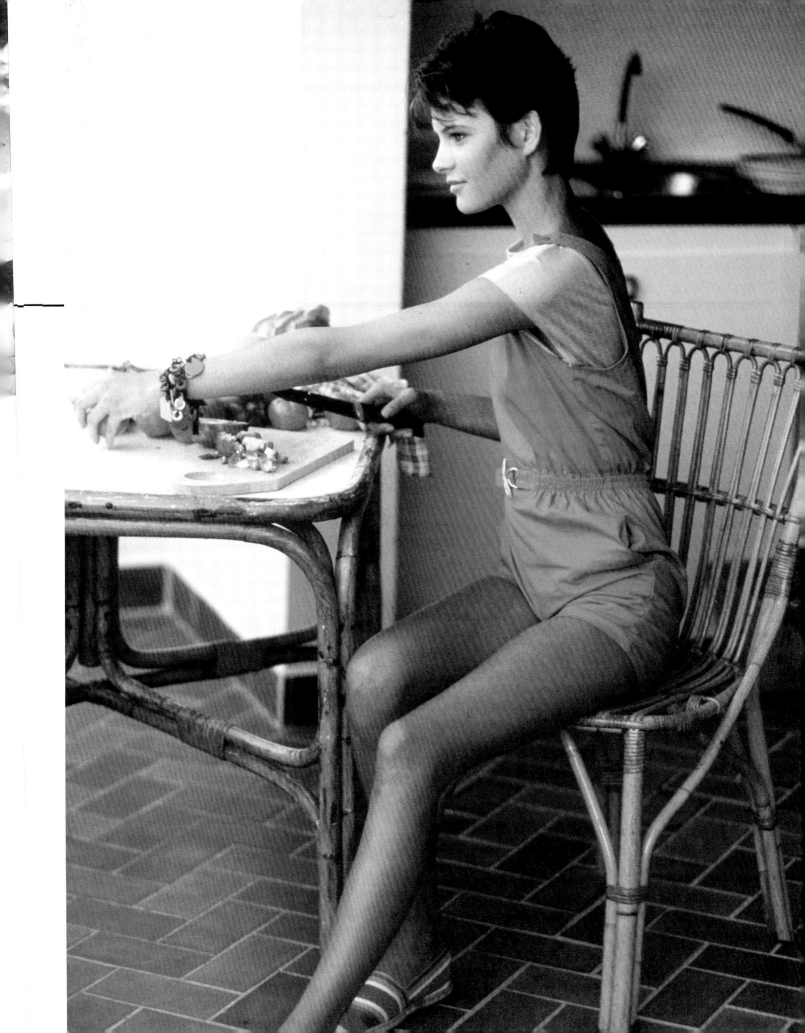

GRILLED TOMATOES (Day 7 Dinner)

Per person:
1   shallot, chopped
1   tablespoon low-calorie oil
1   generous pinch basil or tarragon
Salt
Freshly ground pepper
1   tomato

Mix all ingredients except tomato into as smooth a mixture as possible.

Cut tomato in half. Place in baking dish, cut side up. Drizzle the oil mixture over each half and broil until soft.

WARM MUSHROOM SALAD (Day 8 Dinner)

6   tablespoons low-calorie margarine
5   cloves garlic, finely chopped
Juice of 1 large lemon
1   teaspoon dried tarragon
1   tablespoon red wine vinegar
Salt and pepper to taste
1   pound mushrooms
Lettuce

Heat margarine to a foam in a heavy skillet. Add all ingredients except mushrooms and lettuce. Cook, stirring, until blended. Add mushrooms, cook 5 minutes, stirring constantly. Remove mushrooms and a little of the liquid, spooning over lettuce leaves on salad plates. Serve while warm.

PEPPERED SWORDFISH STEAKS (Day 8 Dinner)

2   teaspoons corn oil
3   swordfish steaks
½   cup dry vermouth
½   cup low-fat yogurt
Salt and pepper to taste
1   teaspoon dry rosemary

Heat 1 teaspoon of oil in heavy skillet. When hot but not boiling, add 2 swordfish steaks and sauté 3 minutes on each side. Keep warm. Add more oil and sauté the other 2 swordfish steaks and keep warm in the oven. Add the vermouth to the skillet and stir. Add yogurt, salt, pepper, and rosemary. Place swordfish on plates and pour sauce over.

Jacki Adams

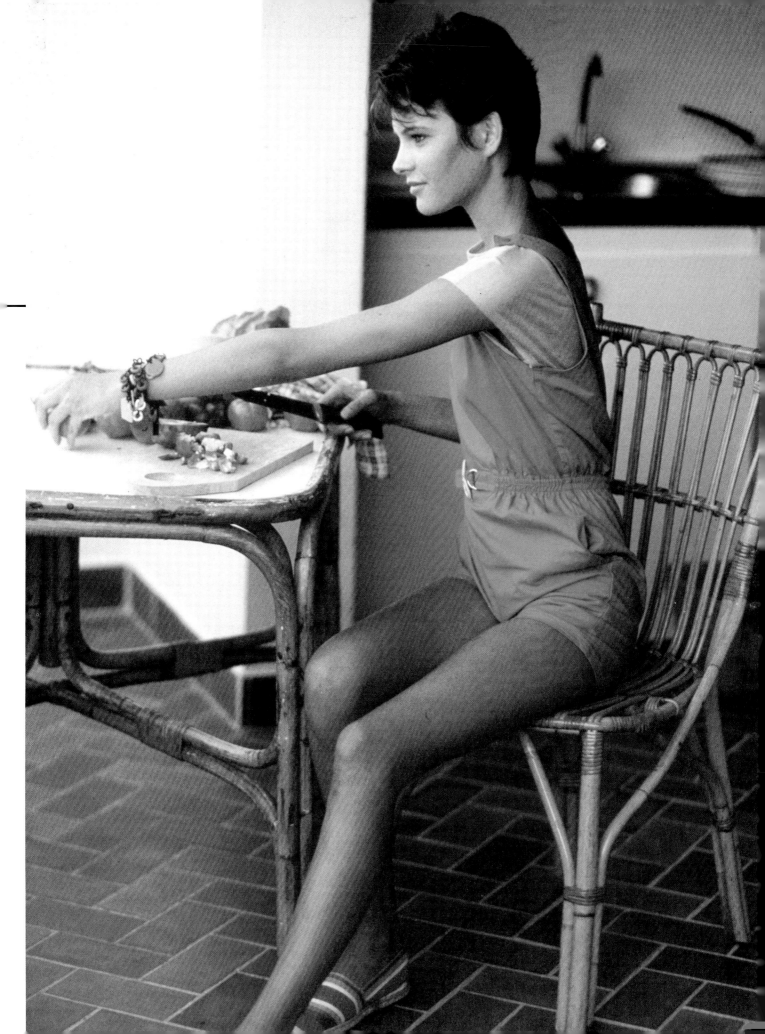

Tomato Coriander Sauce for Spinach Mold

1   cup fresh coriander leaves
¼   cup fresh lime juice or Realime juice
2   peeled cloves garlic
1   cup tomatoes, peeled and seeded
½   teaspoon salt
¾   teaspoon chopped fresh ginger
⅓   cup safflower oil
⅔   cup water

Put all ingredients except the oil into a bowl and mash into a paste. Keep blending as you slowly add the oil with the water. Taste. If needed, add a bit of low-calorie sweetener. Allow to set at room temperature. Spoon over Spinach Mold.

BLACKENED FISH (Day 2 Dinner)

1   fillet (4 ounces) red snapper (or any non-oily fish) per person, seasoned with freshly ground black pepper, a very little chili powder, thyme, white pepper, cayenne
Melted margarine
1 large shrimp per person
Sweet paprika

Heat a heavy iron skillet until almost smoking. Dip seasoned fish fillets in melted margarine and place on hot skillet. Cook about 3 to 5 minutes on each side until cooked but not dry.

Place fillets in a pan, top each with a shrimp dipped in the sauce (recipe below). Sprinkle with sweet paprika and briefly broil in hot oven, about 3 minutes.

Sauce for Blackened Fish (Day 2 Dinner)

1   teaspoon unsalted diet margarine
½   cup minced onion
1   teaspoon minced garlic
3   tablespoons chili powder
¼   cup white wine
2   egg yolks
3   tablespoons clarified butter*
2   teaspoon lemon juice
Salt and pepper

Melt unsalted margarine. Add onion and garlic and cook until limp and transparent. Do not brown. Stir in chili powder and cook another minute over low flame. Keep stirring with wooden spoon.

Deglaze pan and add white wine.

Purée mixture in blender. Pour into a bowl and add 2 egg yolks.

Place bowl over boiling water in a pan. Beat with whisk until mixture forms a continuous ribbon when dribbled from a spoon.

Remove from heat, add clarified butter* in a stream until sauce looks like hollandaise. Add lemon juice, salt and pepper to taste.

ORANGE CABBAGE (Day 2 Dinner)

1   medium cabbage
½   orange
2   cups orange juice

Slice cabbage as for cole slaw. Grate the peel of half an orange and combine with orange juice in a heavy skillet. Heat to a boil. Add the cabbage, cover and allow to cook until just tender. Remove with slotted spoon and serve hot.

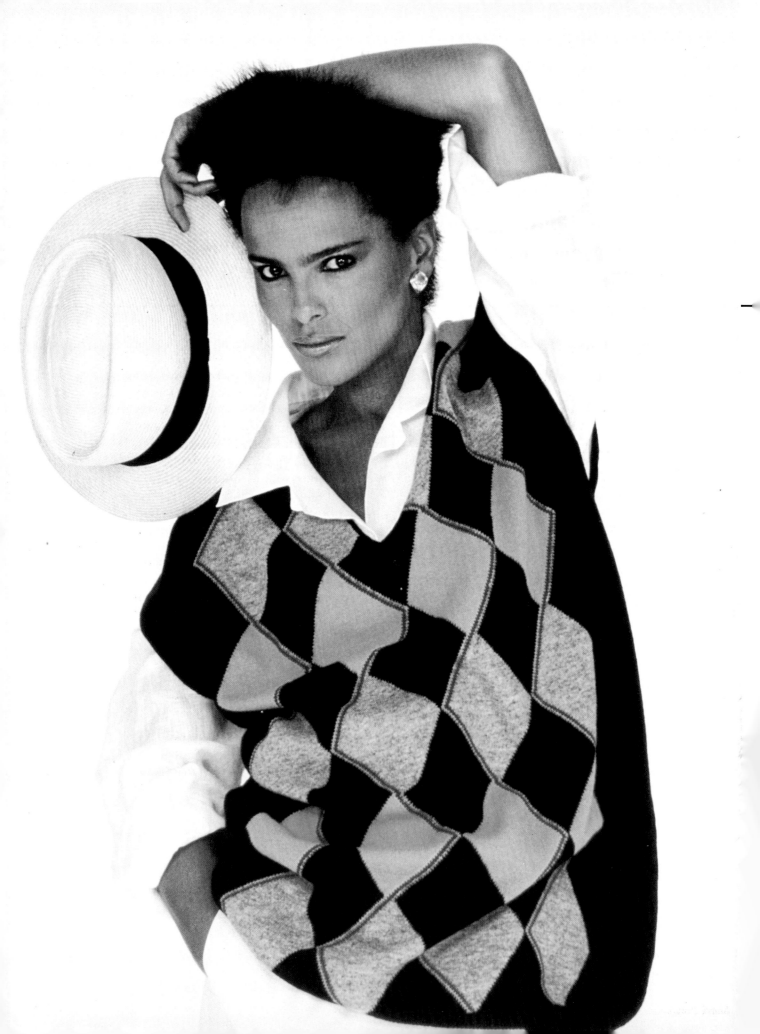

STIR-FRY SPINACH (Day 3 Dinner)

1   teaspoon finely chopped garlic, wilted in
1   teaspoon sesame oil
¼   cup soy sauce
6   cups fresh, shredded spinach, stems removed

Add the soy sauce to wilted garlic and oil in very hot skillet or wok. Turn heat down and simmer 3 minutes. Add shredded spinach to the pan and stir rapidly until spinach is limp. Add salt if needed.

Remove from pan with slotted spoon and serve at once.

STEAMED CHICKEN SANDWICHES (Day 3 Dinner)

7   ounces boned chicken breasts
¾   cup peeled raw shrimp
3   teaspoons finely chopped scallions
2   teaspoons egg whites (from egg whites used to make sauce)
2   teaspoons arrowroot
2   teaspoons sherry
3   tablespoons water
2   pinches salt
4   large lettuce leaves

Reserve ½ chicken breast. Slice remainder into 8 3-inch squares about ¼-inch thick. Finely chop the remaining chicken and the shrimp. Stir in the scallions and egg whites. Add sherry, water and salt. Stir. Set aside for stuffing.

Dust one side of each square with arrowroot. Place 2 tablespoons of stuffing mixture on each of four squares and top with other squares, arrowroot side down.

Blanch lettuce leaves in boiling water for 30 seconds.

Wrap each chicken sandwich in a lettuce leaf, then steam for 10 to 15 minutes or until done.

Sauce for Steamed Chicken Sandwiches

½ cup skimmed chicken broth
8 small mushrooms, sliced
¼ teaspoon salt
1 teaspoon arrowroot
2 egg whites (less 2 teaspoons used in chicken)

Bring chicken broth, mushrooms and salt to a boil. In a small bowl, mix arrowroot and 2 tablespoons of the chicken broth and stir to dissolve. Add this mixture to broth and simmer about 2 minutes until sauce thickens. Remove from heat. Drizzle egg whites into the sauce, stirring constantly with a whisk.
Pour sauce over the steamed chicken sandwiches. Serve at once.

TRINI SALAD (Day 4 Dinner)

4 ripe tomatoes, seeded and diced
½ ball low-fat mozzarella, diced
2 handfuls fresh basil leaves

Mix all ingredients together and stir with oilless dressing, flavored this time with basil.

SALT CHICKEN (Day 4 Dinner)

1 3-pound roasting chicken
Lots of tarragon and rosemary
2 pounds kosher salt
1 egg white

Preheat oven to 350° F. Stuff chicken with herbs. Make a paste of kosher salt and egg white. Coat the chicken with the paste and bake on a rack in the oven for 1½ hours. Remove chicken from oven, crack the shell, remove with the skin and discard.

HERB BRAISED FISH (Day 5 Dinner)

1   thinly sliced onion
1   thinly sliced small leek
1   sliced carrot
1   bay leaf
½   cup mushrooms, sliced
1   halibut (or similar non-oily white fish)
Salt
½   cup clam juice
¾   cup dry white or red wine
1   cup yogurt or crème fraîche*

Preheat oven to 375° F.

Place the sliced vegetables in a baking dish. Place the fish (with or without head and tail) in dish on top of vegetables. Pour the clam juice and wine over the fish. Sprinkle with salt to taste. Cover and bake for ½ hour or longer, depending on the size of the fish. Remove from oven and skin fish. Place on serving platter and keep warm.

Bring sauce to boil and cook until it is reduced to ⅓ its volume. Strain, return to pan. Add yogurt or crème fraîche* and gently heat until thickened.

Pour sauce over fish and serve.

TOMATO BOUILLON (Day 5 Dinner)

5   cups beef bouillon
½   cup sherry
2   beaten egg whites plus 1 egg shell
1   pound soup bones
4   stalks celery including leaves, chopped
2   leeks, chopped
1   medium onion, chopped
1   carrot, chopped
5   ripe tomatoes, chopped
1   package low-calorie sweetener
Salt and a few grinds fresh black pepper

Cook all ingredients at a very slow boil for 1 hour. Strain into a bowl, pressing out the fluid. Strain again through a cheesecloth. (I make a lot of this in the summer and freeze it in ice trays. Then I store the cubes in plastic bags for future use.)

SPINACH WITH ONION POWDER (Day 5 Dinner)

1   box frozen chopped spinach, cooked and drained
½   teaspoon onion powder
1   tablespoon low-calorie margarine
Salt to taste

Stir onion powder and margarine into spinach. Add a pinch of salt and serve.

RAW VEGETABLE SALAD (Day 6 Dinner)

Cauliflower flowerets
Thinly sliced zucchini
Sliced cucumber
Broccoli
Thinly sliced carrots
Garlic
Oilless dressing*
1   tablespoon crème fraîche* or low-fat yogurt

Combine vegetables in a salad bowl that has been rubbed with garlic. Toss the vegetables in oilless dressing* to which has been added 1 tablespoon crème fraîche* or plain low-fat yogurt.

GARLIC BAKED SHRIMP (Day 6 Dinner)

1   cup white wine
½   cup corn oil
3   cloves garlic, finely chopped
1   teaspoon salt
Pinch of cayenne
2   pounds peeled large shrimps

Combine wine, oil, garlic, salt, cayenne. Add shrimp and mix.
    Heat broiler for 10 minutes.
    Place shrimp on broiler pan and broil 5 minutes on each side, basting frequently with marinade. Allow eight shrimps per person.

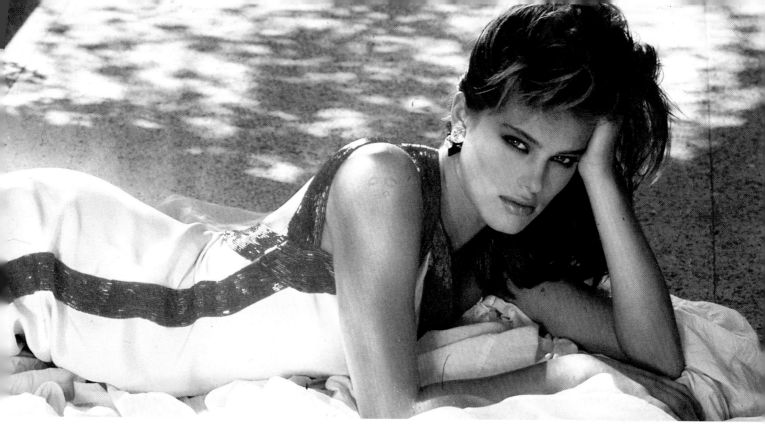

Renée Simonsen

CRUDITÉS (Day 7 Dinner)

Take a whole cucumber, a ripe tomato, a whole zucchini, one carrot, a bunch of celery from which the outer stalks have been removed, and any other raw vegetable in season. Cut into pieces or sticks.

Serve as first course with salt and lemon pepper.

BASS IN FOIL (Day 7 Dinner)

8   tablespoons softened diet margarine
2   tablespoons minced parsley
3   cloves of garlic, minced
2   tablespoons fresh tarragon or rosemary
2   tablespoons of minced onion or shallots
1   3-pound bass, with head and tail
Juice of 1 lemon
½   teaspoon dried thyme
2   bay leaves
2   sprigs parsley
Salt
Fresh ground pepper
6   scrubbed mussels (optional)
6   peeled raw shrimp (optional)
6   clams (optional)
3   tablespoons white part of fennel, chopped (optional)

Heat oven to 400° F.

With a whisk, blend and then beat the margarine, parsley, garlic, tarragon or rosemary, and onion or shallots into a paste. Wash fish with water, drain, and pat dry with paper towels.

Sprinkle fish with lemon juice. Place thyme, bay leaf and parsley inside fish. Sprinkle with salt and pepper. Brush with half the margarine mixture.

Place a large piece of foil in a shallow baking dish. Rub the remaining margarine mixture on the inside of the foil. Now place the fish, the shellfish (optional), and chopped fennel (optional), on the foil. Seal the foil into a bag.

Bake for 50 minutes. Slice bag open and remove fish to serving dish. Pour juices over fish before serving.

GRILLED TOMATOES (Day 7 Dinner)

Per person:
1   shallot, chopped
1   tablespoon low-calorie oil
1   generous pinch basil or tarragon
Salt
Freshly ground pepper
1   tomato

Mix all ingredients except tomato into as smooth a mixture as possible.

Cut tomato in half. Place in baking dish, cut side up. Drizzle the oil mixture over each half and broil until soft.

WARM MUSHROOM SALAD (Day 8 Dinner)

6   tablespoons low-calorie margarine
5   cloves garlic, finely chopped
Juice of 1 large lemon
1   teaspoon dried tarragon
1   tablespoon red wine vinegar
Salt and pepper to taste
1   pound mushrooms
Lettuce

Heat margarine to a foam in a heavy skillet. Add all ingredients except mushrooms and lettuce. Cook, stirring, until blended. Add mushrooms, cook 5 minutes, stirring constantly. Remove mushrooms and a little of the liquid, spooning over lettuce leaves on salad plates. Serve while warm.

PEPPERED SWORDFISH STEAKS (Day 8 Dinner)

2   teaspoons corn oil
3   swordfish steaks
½   cup dry vermouth
½   cup low-fat yogurt
Salt and pepper to taste
1   teaspoon dry rosemary

Heat 1 teaspoon of oil in heavy skillet. When hot but not boiling, add 2 swordfish steaks and sauté 3 minutes on each side. Keep warm. Add more oil and sauté the other 2 swordfish steaks and keep warm in the oven. Add the vermouth to the skillet and stir. Add yogurt, salt, pepper, and rosemary. Place swordfish on plates and pour sauce over.

Jacki Adams

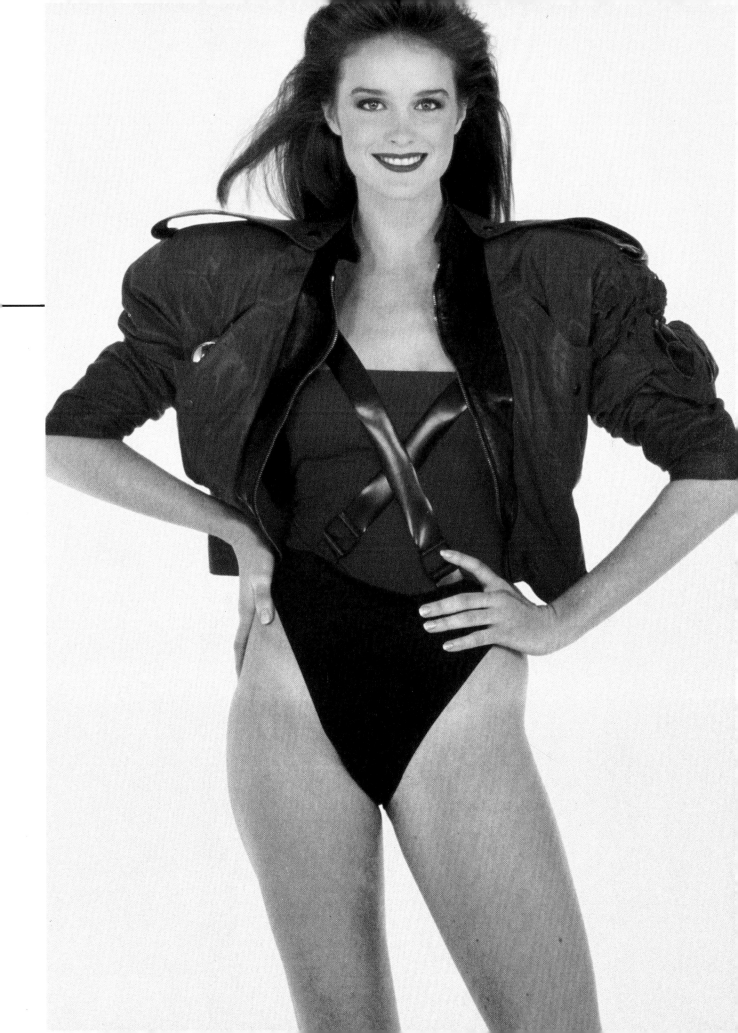

POACHED BASS (Day 9 Dinner)

1   3-pound bass (have it cleaned, leav-
    ing backbone in. Sprinkle it lightly
    with salt and wrap in cheesecloth).
5   cups water
1   cup dry white wine
1   large onion, chopped
1   carrot, sliced
1   bay leaf
1   handful celery leaves
3   sprigs parsley
1   large tomato, chopped
Pinch of dried thyme
1   dozen dried green peppercorns
Coriander

Place all ingredients except fish and coriander in a baking dish. Cover. Bring to a
boil and taste for seasoning. Simmer
slowly for ½ hour. Add the wrapped fish.
Liquid should just cover fish; add water if
needed. Simmer for 25 minutes longer.

Remove baking dish from flame and
let fish cool in the liquid. When ready to
serve, transfer to a platter being careful
not to break the fish.

Strain liquid over the fish and sprinkle
with ground or dried coriander.

CHINESE CHICKEN (Day 10 Dinner)

1   3-pound roasting chicken
Sea salt
4   cups canned low-calorie chicken broth
2   cups oriental soy sauce
4   scallions, chopped
4   slices fresh ginger
4   tablespoons medium-dry sherry

Wash chicken and dry thoroughly. Rub
inside with sea salt.

Combine all other ingredients in a
deep saucepan. Bring to a boil. Add
chicken and boil gently for 5 minutes.
Reduce heat and simmer, covered, for 15
minutes. Turn chicken, simmer for 15
minutes longer. Turn chicken, simmer for
10 minutes longer. Turn again and simmer until done, which should be only a
few more minutes. Optional: now brush
chicken with corn oil and brown under
the broiler.

Slice chicken. Serve at room temperature with the sauce.

WATERCRESS PURÉE (Day 11 Dinner)

1   quart low-calorie chicken broth
1   tablespoon sea salt
6   bunches watercress (leaves only)

Bring broth to a boil; add salt and watercress leaves. Simmer 5 minutes. Remove watercress; drain and blot dry with paper towel. Purée in a blender, adding a little broth as needed. Do not allow it to become too liquid.

BAKED SALMON (Day 12 Dinner)

1   tablespoon low-calorie margarine
1   cup finely sliced carrots
⅓   cup chopped shallots
½   cup diced fennel, plus a pinch of fennel seeds
1   teaspoon dried thyme
3   sprigs parsley
1   cup white wine
⅓   cup bottled clam broth
Salt
6   4-ounce salmon steaks
3   egg yolks, beaten
2   tablespoons capers, drained

Heat margarine in large skillet. Sauté carrots, shallots, fennel, thyme and parsley for 3 minutes. Add white wine and clam broth.

Add salted salmon steaks, placing on top of vegetable mixture. Cover tightly with foil. Bake in preheated 350° F. oven for 15 minutes. Remove fish and keep warm on heated platter.

Strain liquid into a saucepan; add 3 beaten egg yolks and beat over low heat until sauce is thick. Stir in well-drained capers. Pour sauce over fish.

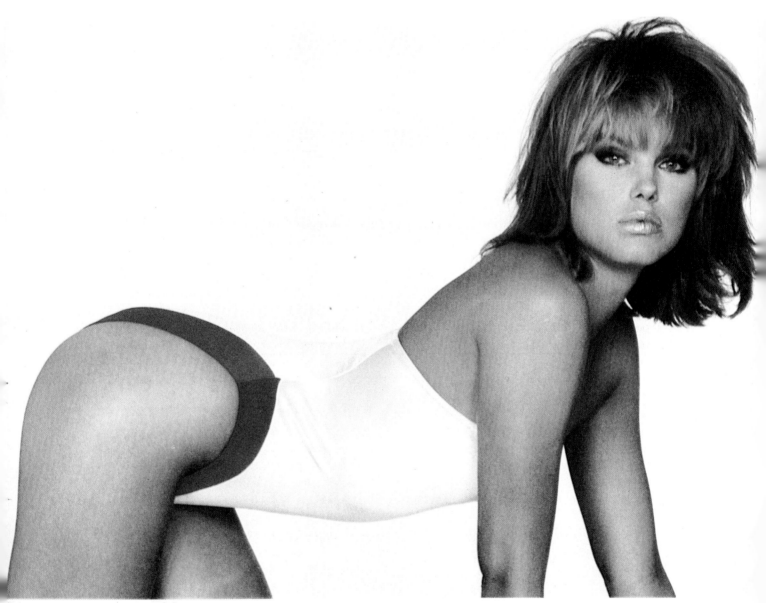

Renée Simonsen

HERBED TOMATO SOUP (Day 13 Dinner)

Canned tomato soup
½ cup basil leaves
1 clove garlic, chopped

Heat soup with other ingredients. Strain.

SAUTÉED SCALLOPS (Day 13 Dinner)

1 pound bay scallops
4 teaspoons low-calorie margarine
1 cup white wine
½ cup chopped shallots
½ teaspoon chopped garlic
¼ teaspoon salt
1 teaspoon powdered fennel
4 tablespoons Pernod
½ teaspoon fennel seeds

Wash scallops in cold water; drain; pat dry with paper towel.

Heat margarine in a heavy skillet. Add all ingredients except scallops. Cook, covered, very slowly for 30 minutes. Add scallops and simmer for 8 minutes. Serve at once.

PURÉED SPINACH (Day 13 Dinner)

1 package frozen chopped spinach
¼ teaspoon onion powder
Salt to taste

Cook spinach for 4 minutes with very little water, onion powder and salt. Drain. Place in blender and purée. Add a little liquid if necessary to make a smooth mixture.

HERB ROASTED CHICKEN (Day 14 Dinner)

1 3-pound roasting chicken
Salt and pepper
Tarragon or herbes de Provence
1 large onion, peeled
1 clove garlic
Corn oil
Paprika

Wash chicken and sprinkle with salt and pepper, tarragon or herbes de Provence, inside and out. Place onion and garlic inside chicken. Brush with corn oil and sprinkle with paprika. Roast in preheated 350° F. oven for 1 hour.

ZUCCHINI MOLD WITH TOMATO SAUCE
(Day 14 Dinner)

3   zucchinis
8   tablespoons low-fat ricotta cheese
1   teaspoon dried basil
8   egg whites, beaten stiff

Boil zucchinis in salted water for 3 minutes. Drain. Purée in blender. Squeeze liquid from zucchinis.

Combine zucchini, ricotta cheese, basil and gently fold in beaten egg whites. Spoon into 4 custard cups. Place cups in a pan; fill pan with water to reach ¾ up the cups. Bake in 350° F. preheated oven until firm, about 20 minutes. Serve at once with tomato sauce.

Tomato Sauce

3   tablespoons corn oil
2   teaspoons Dijon mustard
2   tablespoons chopped tarragon and/
    or parsley
1   tablespoon chopped scallions
6   crushed coriander seeds
Salt and pepper
3   cups raw seeded tomatoes, diced

Mix all ingredients together except for the tomatoes. Beat with a whisk. Add salt and pepper. Add tomatoes. Mix and heat. Pour over zucchini molds or serve separately.

CRÈME FRAÎCHE

2   tablespoons low-fat sour cream
2   tablespoons heavy cream

Mix together ingredients. Cover and let stand for 12 hours. Refrigerate 24 more hours before using.

CLARIFIED BUTTER

Heat butter in a small saucepan over medium heat. Skim off the foam as it rises and keep skimming until no more foam is formed. When pouring the butter, make sure you leave any milky residue in the pan.

OILLESS SALAD DRESSING

1   teaspoon finely chopped garlic
2   tablespoons scallions or onions, finely chopped
1   tablespoon dried mint, tarragon and basil
½   teaspoon salt
4   tablespoons French mustard
2   tablespoons lemon juice (or a bit more if you like)

Crush garlic, scallions and herbs and mix together with enough salt to form a paste. Gradually add mustard, beating with a whisk. Add one ice cube and blend in lemon juice slowly. Store in refrigerator.

You can make this dressing any flavor you desire by using just one herb such as basil, tarragon, dill, a combination, or none at all. If fresh herbs are not available, use dried.

ANOTHER LOW-CALORIE SALAD DRESSING

5   tablespoons low-fat ricotta cheese
2   tablespoons balsamic vinegar or red wine vinegar
2   teaspoons Dijon mustard
1   teaspoon herbes de Provence
½   teaspoon salt
1   grind of black peppercorns

Mix all ingredients together in a bowl with one cube of ice.

As in other dressing, use any herbs (fresh or dried) that suit your fancy.

OILLESS VINAIGRETTE

To the recipe for oilless dressing, add 1 tablespoon chopped onion, 1 tablespoon chopped green pepper, 1 tablespoon chopped parsley and 1 tablespoon chopped hard-boiled egg. Stir all ingredients into dressing.

This sauce is great over cold asparagus or cold cooked artichokes, and has very few calories.

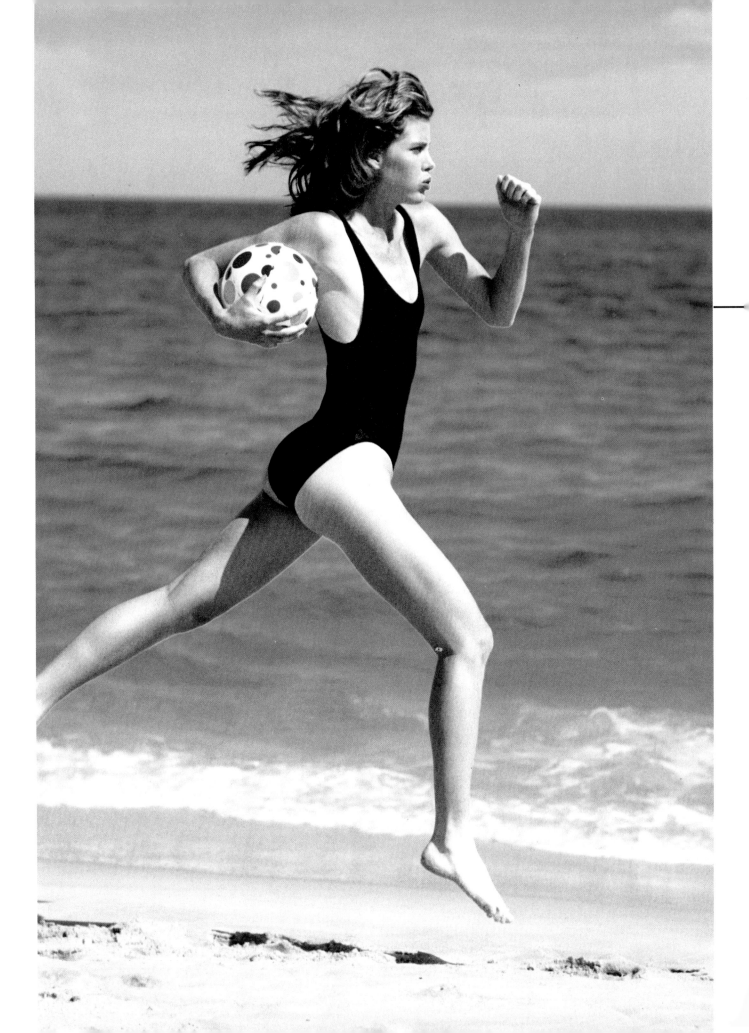

THE FORD MODELS' QUICK SHAPE-UP EXERCISE PLAN

Models are lean, smooth, and firmly packed, and there are few who don't follow a daily exercise program because their careers depend on having great bodies.

The health clubs in New York are thronged with Ford models working out on the machines and participating in aerobics classes. Central Park is full of them, running along the paths early morning or evening, sometimes in packs of six or eight. Madison Avenue finds them striding down the street, their big bags or one-pound weights in their hands, hurrying to their bookings. A few of our models bicycle everywhere they go in New York, through the heavy traffic, behind buses and around parks (a suicidal habit to my mind). Go to any pool in midtown Manhattan and you'll find Ford models swimming laps. In their apartments, many more are doing floor exercises, working out on rowing machines, jumping on mini-trampolines, practicing yoga. All because they know exercise is an essential ingredient of good looks as well as good health.

TIME TO SHAPE UP

This chapter is dedicated to you, the great majority of American women who aren't in *all* that bad shape, who aren't *really* fat, but whose bodies sure could use help. Help is here but you must be ready to spend about half an hour a day—at least three times a week—to firm your body. If our models can fit this small amount of time into their busy schedules and I can fit it into mine, you can, too. Once you start the program, you will see an enormous difference in only a few weeks. It is designed to get you in shape fast and then keep you there.

Combined with the Ford Models' Quick Shape-up Diet, this program will help you *remake* your body and change your life. You will not only develop a lean, smooth body like our models, but you will have energy you never felt before.

It doesn't really matter what form of exercise you get, as long as you get it and do it vigorously enough to raise your heart rate to around 70 to 80 percent of its maximum capacity. This will improve the workings of your heart and lungs, strengthen your bones, relieve tension, and burn off calories. That means "aerobic" exercise for at least 15 minutes. So, if you want to jump rope or ride a bike, fine; whatever appeals to you. I personally have tried many varieties of exercise, including aerobic dancing, which I never could master because I am not well coordinated and I was even evicted from one class because I was always going the wrong way!

It's not smart to go against your own inclinations, because if you hate what you're doing, you'll quit. Make your choice but choose *something*.

The Ford Models' exercise program was devised for our models by our health-minded daughter, Lacey. If you follow it, it will do for you what it has done for her, her mother and a whole generation of beautiful women you see in magazines and on the television screen. One major attribute is that it isn't boring—there's plenty of variety and it's easy to tell what each exercise is doing for what part of you.

We give the program to models who have good bodies but need to be firmed up. We hand it to others who have gained five or ten pounds they hadn't planned on and need to get them off fast. And we give it to those who have parts that need shaping.

The Ford Models' Quick Shape-up Exercise Plan may seem vigorous—it is. Exercise won't do any good if it isn't vigorous. Start slowly, especially if aerobic exercise is new to you. You don't have to conquer the exercises that seem difficult all at once. You don't have to be perfect. What you have to be is persistent and consistent. If you are really out of shape, do only one or two of each routine to start and work up to the required number.

FORD MODELS' QUICK SHAPE-UP EXERCISE PLAN

Before you exercise, take a hot shower to loosen up your muscles. Then begin every session with some simple stretches. Now move into the aerobics for 15 to 20 minutes, without stopping between exercises. Make sure you get your heart and lungs pumping hard enough to speed up your metabolism. (Remember, as with any exercise plan, to get medical clearance from your doctor before you begin.)

To calculate what your heart rate should be during aerobic exercise, use this easy formula and then check your pulse at intervals during the session to be sure you are not exceeding that number:

Take the number 220, subtract your age, then take 80 percent of that number. For example, if you are 25: 220 minus 25 equals 195. Eighty percent of 195 equals 156. So, 156 is about what your heart rate should be during your exercise session.

Continue the aerobics for the full 15 or 20 minutes, slowing down or speeding up according to your ability and pulse rate. Run through all the exercises and then start again until your time is up.

The easiest way to take your pulse is to put your fingertips on the artery in your neck, just beneath your jaw. Count the number of throbs or pulses in 15 seconds, then multiply by 4. That's your pulse rate.

The next step in the Ford Models' Quick Shape-up Exercise Plan is exercises for specific parts of you. You need them all for toning and firming, and more of some of them if you have problem areas.

FORD MODELS AEROBICS

SLOW
JOG

- Stand straight, holding abdomen tight.
- Jog slowly in place, landing on your toes and then touching your whole foot to the floor.

- Pump your arms as you jog.

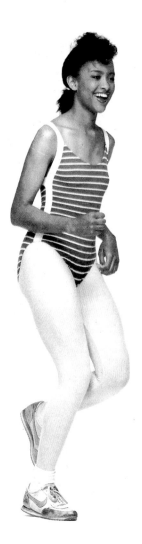

The model for the aerobics sequence on pages 188–200 is Karen Williams.

SHOULDER
ROLLS

ur sides, feet

ur ears, then

a continuous

- Reverse directions.
- Continue without stopping for 30 seconds in each direction.

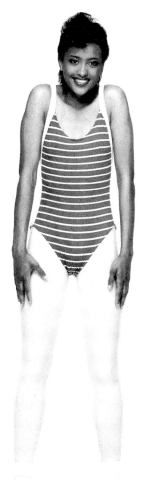

CEILING CLIMB

- Stand, feet apart.
- Reach your right arm up as high as possible while reaching down with your left arm. Stretch hard, feeling the pull in your waist.
- Reverse, stretching your left arm up and your right arm down.
- Continue, alternating arms.

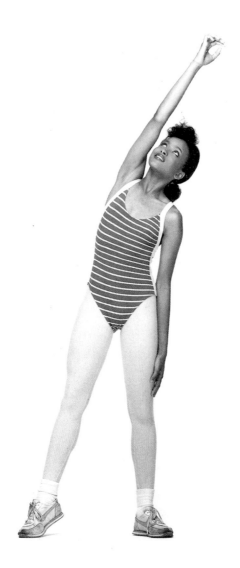

TORSO
TWISTS

- Stand with feet apart, knees slightly bent. Tuck pelvis under, holding abdomen tight.

- Swing both arms loosely from side to side, allowing your whole torso to twist around as you swing and following with your head.

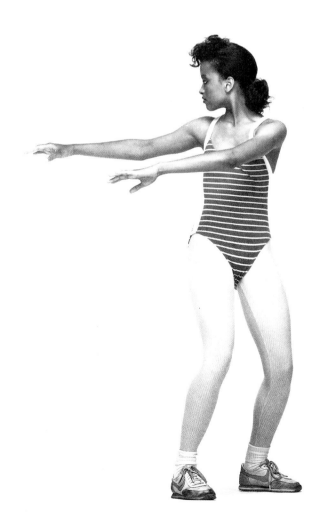

THE MINI
CANCAN

- Stand, arms straight out to the sides.
- Jump on both feet, then hop onto your left foot while raising your right knee.
- Land on both feet.
- Hop on one foot, kicking the other as high as possible.
- Land on both feet.
- Continue sequence for one minute, alternating legs.

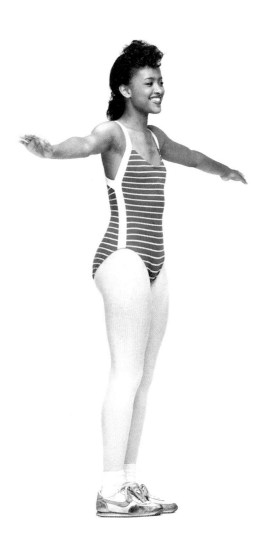

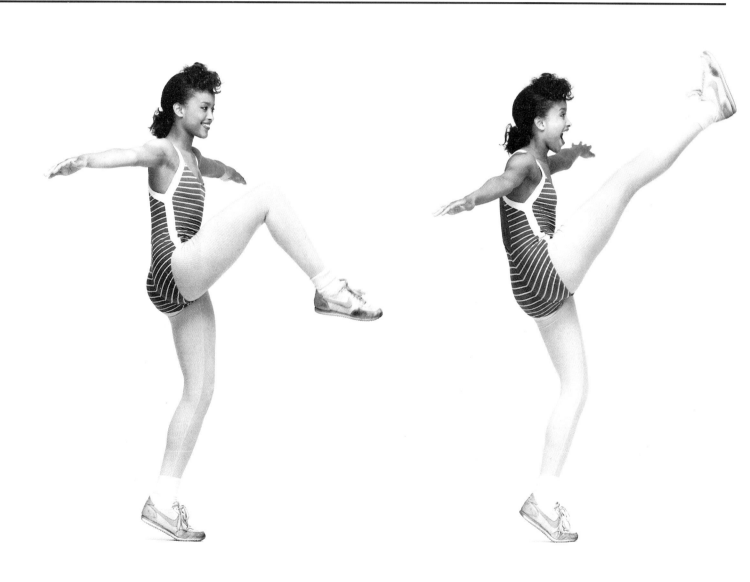

THE SCISSORS

- Stand with feet apart, toes pointed out. Tuck pelvis under. Stretch arms out to the sides.
- Swing arms forward, crossing them at the wrists, and at the same time, bend your knees outward, squatting with straight back and keeping heels flat on the floor.
- Stand up, raising arms out to the sides again.

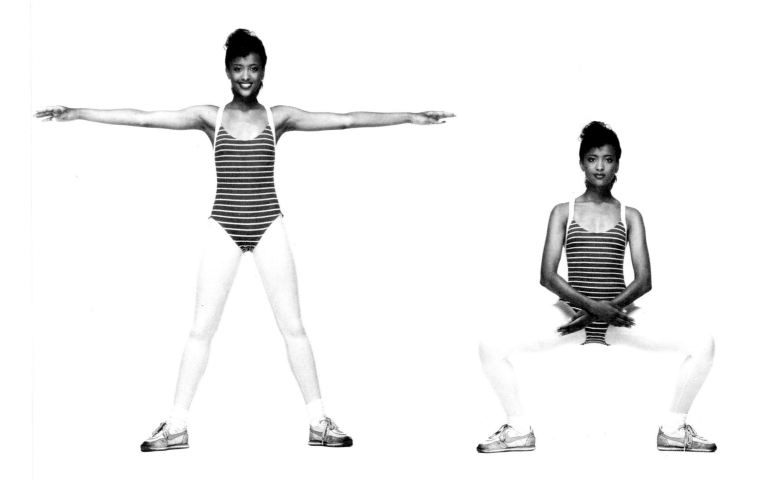

BALLET HOP

- Stand with knees bent, toes pointed out to the sides, one ankle crossed over the other.
- Jump up and land in the same position, reversing your crossed feet.

- Jump continuously for about one minute.

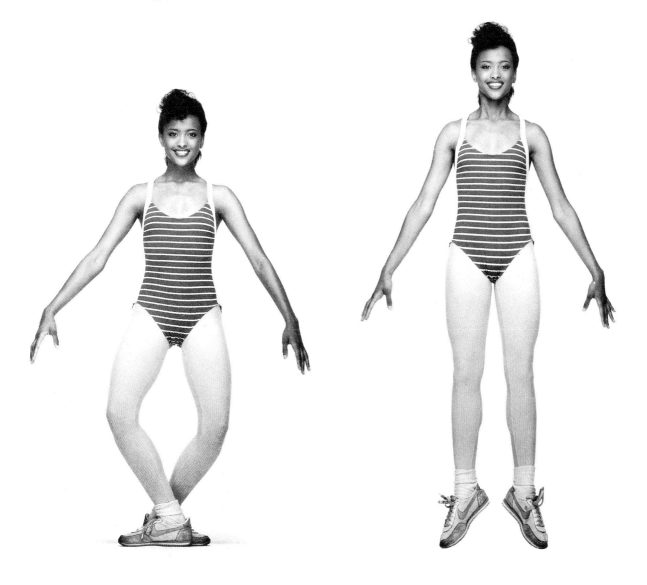

TWIST AND
BEND

- Stand with feet apart, toes pointed slightly out, arms stretched above your head.
- Twist to the right. Reach up and stretch down to touch both hands to your right foot. Move briskly.

- Straighten up.
- Do the same to the left side.
- Continue, alternating sides.

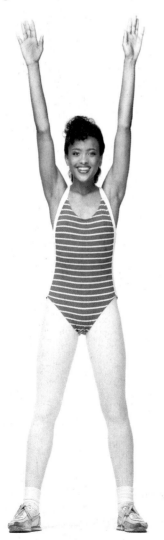

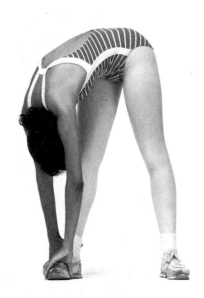

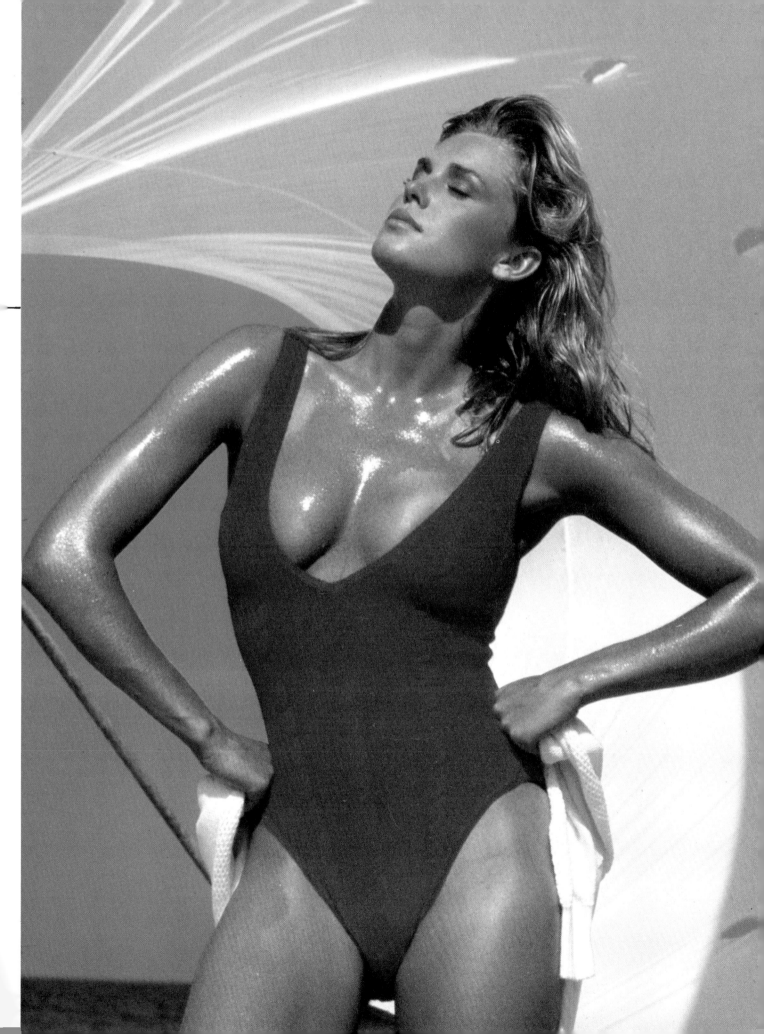

FOR THE WAISTLINE

TORSO
TWIST

- Sit on the floor, right leg folded in, left leg folded back.
- Bend elbows and raise arms to shoulder level, palms down.
- Twist torso down toward your left knee, pointing your chin over your left shoulder.

- Swing elbows back toward right knee and bend forward bringing your elbows to your sides. Fall to your hands and touch your nose to the floor above your knee.
- Repeat 20 times, then reverse legs and repeat on the other side 20 times.

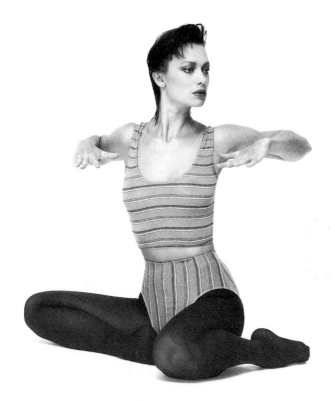

The model for the waistline exercises on pages 202–207 is Vibeke.

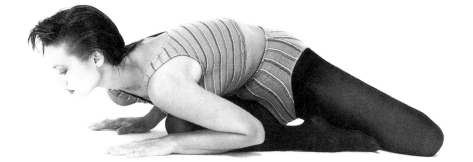

THE
HALLELUJAH

1. • Stand with feet apart, toes pointing out, pelvis tucked under. Bend elbows at your sides.
   • Bend knees outward.
   • Push both arms over your head, stretching hard, as you straighten your legs.
   • Repeat 20 times.
2. • Stand in the same position.
   • Bend knees outward.
   • Leaning your upper torso to the right, push your arms over your head as you straighten your legs.
   • Return to starting position.
   • Repeat 20 times, then do the same on the left side.

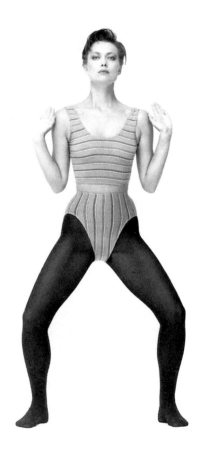

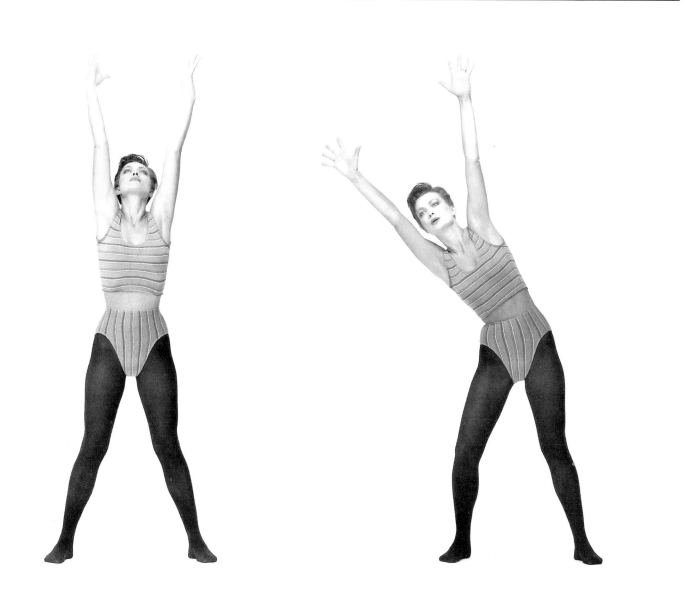

AROUND
THE BEND

1. • Stand with legs apart, right foot turned slightly out.
   • Cross your hands behind your back as high as possible.
   • Turn torso *to the right* and bend over with a straight back, head up.
   • Now drop head to right knee, rounding your back, and bounce three times.
   • Raise torso to flat-back position over your right foot and return to starting position.
2. • Stand in starting position, facing forward, hands crossed high behind your back.
   • Head up and back straight, bend *forward.*
   • Drop head to knee level, rounding your back, and bounce three times.
   • Raise torso to flat-back position and return to starting position.
3. • Repeat as in 1. on the *left* side.
   • Repeat the entire sequence 10 times.

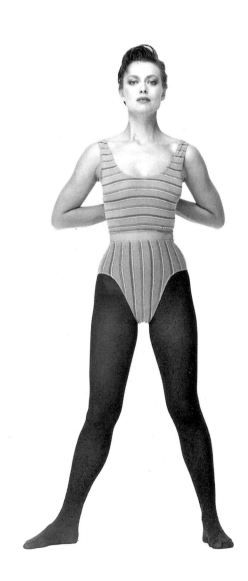

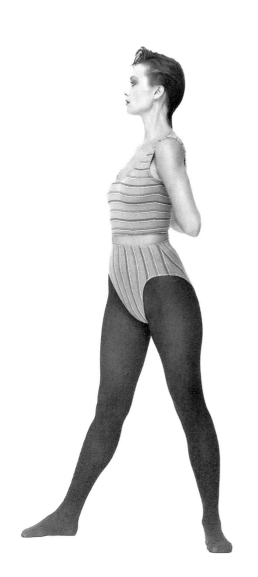

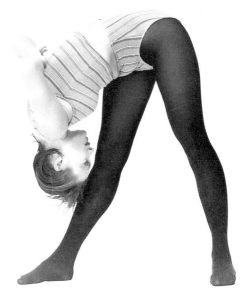

FOR THE ABDOMEN

SIDE
WINDER

- Lie on your back, hands clasped behind your neck. Raise your legs, crossing them at the ankles, knees bent and out.
- Raise your upper torso off the floor.
- Twist your torso to the right toward your right knee. Hold.

- Twist to the left. Hold.
- Return to center with torso raised. Lower body slowly.
- Repeat whole sequence 20 times.

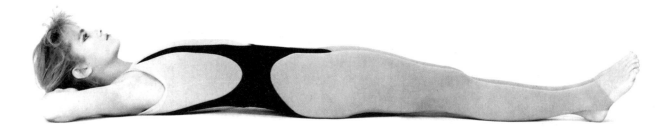

The model for the abdomen exercises on pages 208–215 and on page 217 is Marlene Bergh.

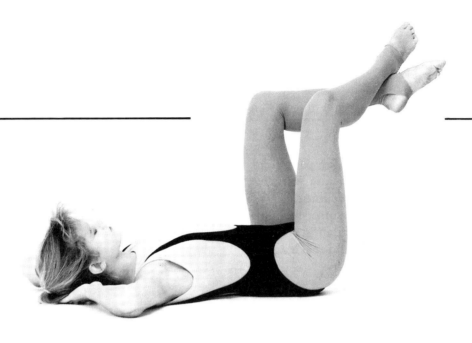

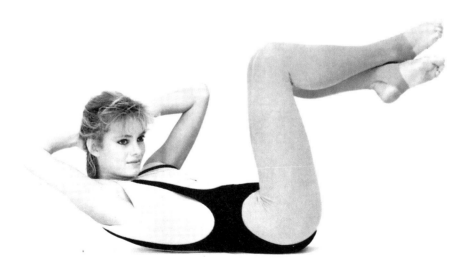

ROLL-UPS

- Sit with back straight, arms and legs straight out in front, feet flexed.
- Lean forward, touch toes, and hold for two counts.

- Now roll back slowly, touching your shoulders to the floor on the count of 8. Hold for two counts.
- Roll up vertebra by vertebra.
- Repeat 10 times.

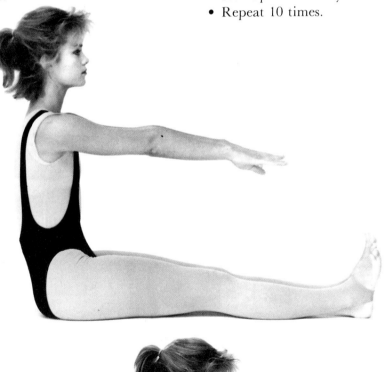

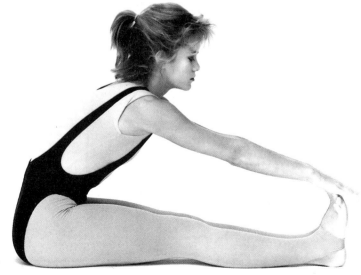

NOTE: If you tend to have back problems or find this difficult, keep your knees
bent and your feet tucked under a sofa.

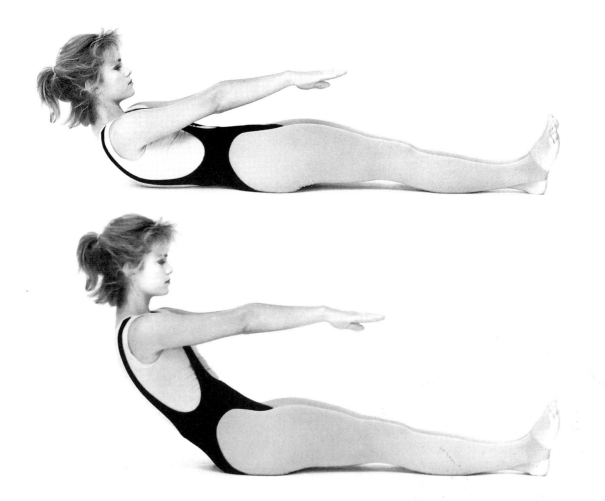

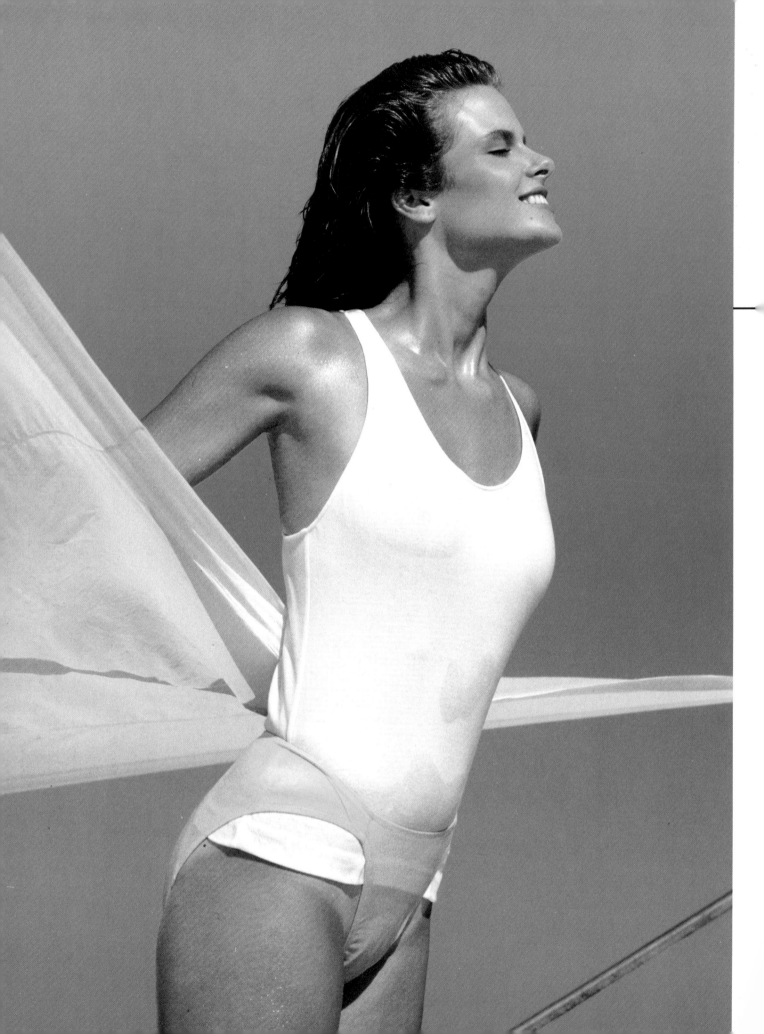

COOL-DOWN

- Lie on your back, arms at your sides. Bend your knees toward your chest.
- Keeping your shoulders flat on the floor, drop your knees to the right, hold for 10 counts.

- Bring knees up and drop them to the left, holding for 10 counts.
- Continue for about one minute.

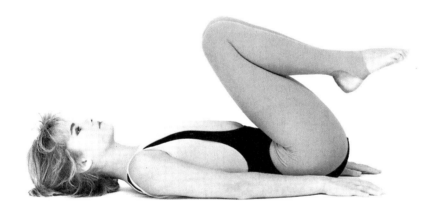

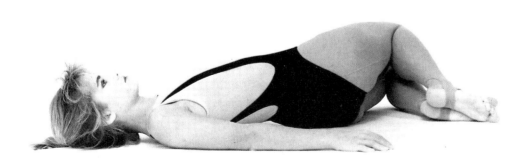

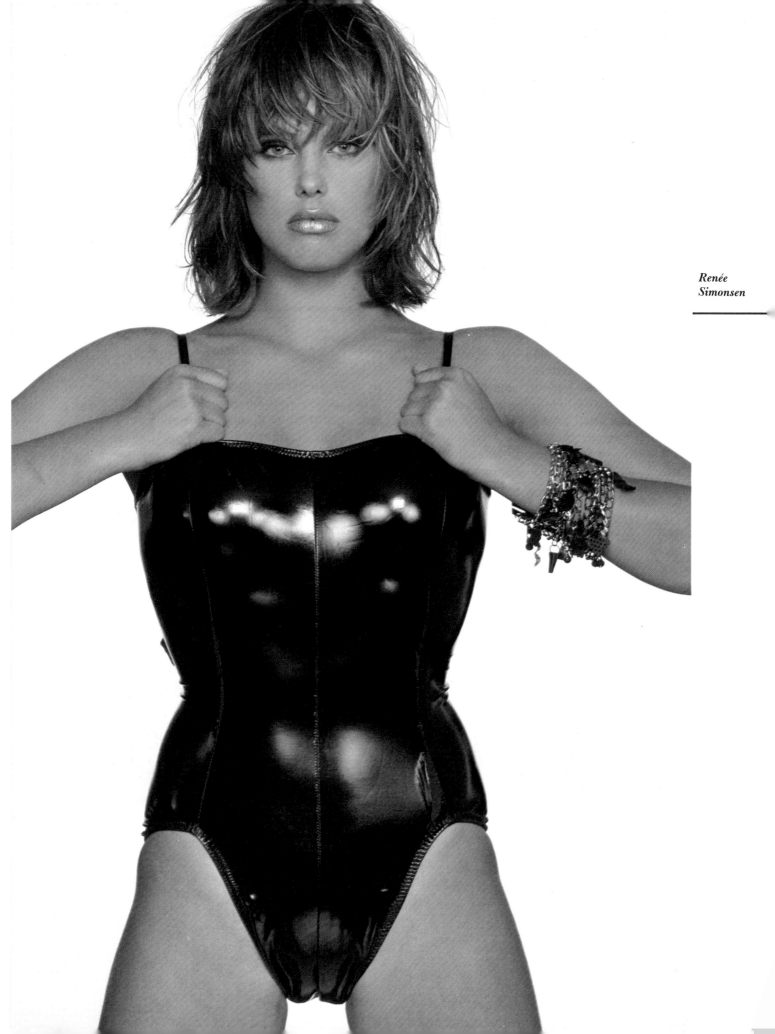

FOR THE LEGS

LAZY LEG STRETCH

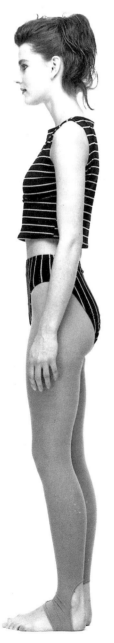

- Stand with feet together.
- Roll down until your hands reach the floor, trying not to bend your knees.
- Hang there (don't bounce) for a count of 20.

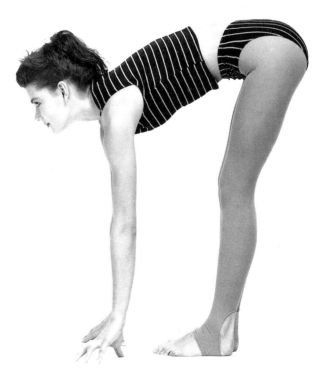

The model for the leg exercises on pages 223–231 is Heidi Schaefer.

KICKBACK

1. • Stand with feet apart. Bend over, letting your knees bend if necessary and place your fingers on the floor just in front of and a little to the sides of your feet.
   • Using your right leg and your fingers for support, kick your *straight* left leg back in a straight line with your back. Keep your foot flexed.
   • Pulse your heel toward the ceiling in quick small movements for 20 counts.

   • Now point your toe and pulse again for 20 counts.
   • Repeat for the right leg.
2. • Bend over in the same position, fingers on the floor.
   • This time, with your weight on right leg and your fingers, *bend* your left leg up at a 90-degree angle.
   • With foot flexed, kick your leg up toward the ceiling 20 times.
   • Repeat with your right leg 20 times.

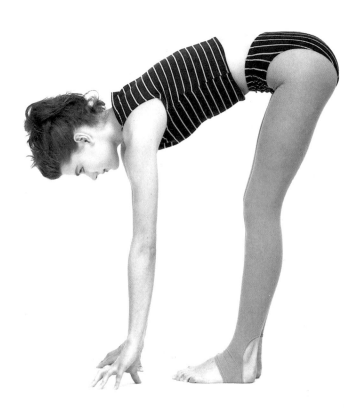

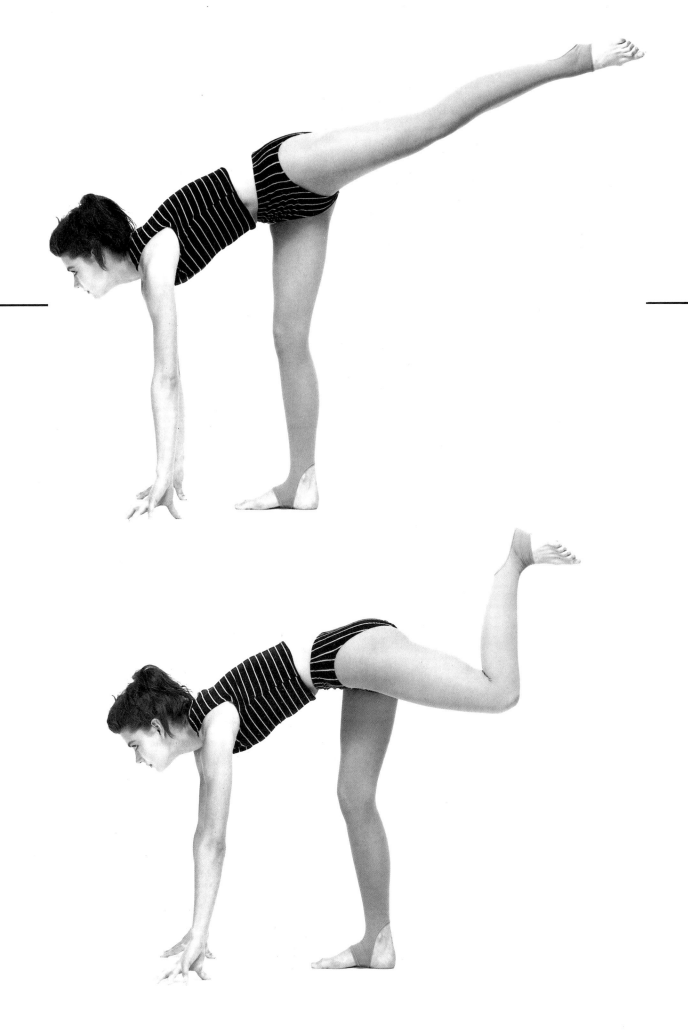

KILLER LEG
CIRCLES

1. • Sit on the floor, back straight, leaning back on your straight arms.
   • Bend your right leg and extend your left leg in front of you about six inches off the floor.
   • With pointed toes, make small circles with your left foot five times in one direction, then five times in the other.

   • With flexed foot, do the same.
   • Repeat with right foot.
2. • In the same position, open your right leg as wide to the side as possible.
   • Make large wide circles with pointed toes, then flexed feet, five times in both directions.
   • Repeat with left leg.

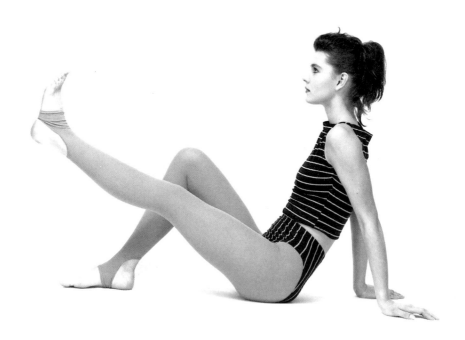

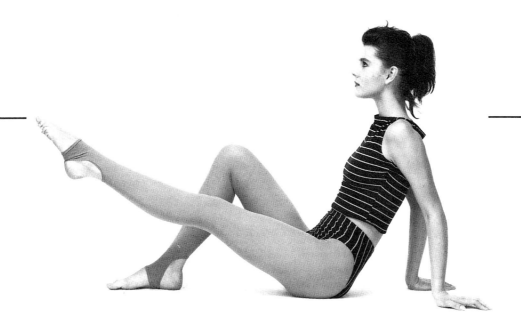

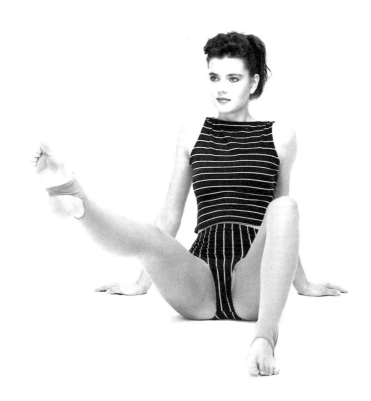

LEG
SWINGS

- Sit with back straight and leaning back on straight arms.
- Bend right knee, foot flat on the floor.
- Bend left leg into your chest, then kick it straight out in front. Swing it out to the side as wide as possible, then back to the front. Bend it into the chest again. Repeat 20 times.
- Switch legs and repeat 20 times.

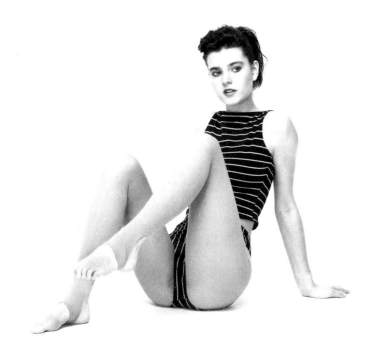

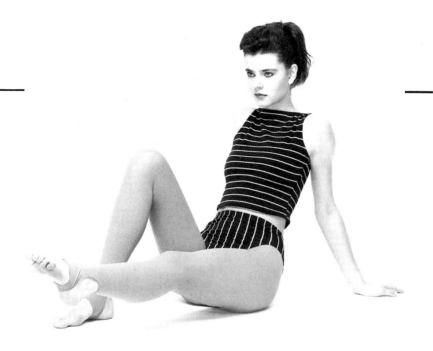

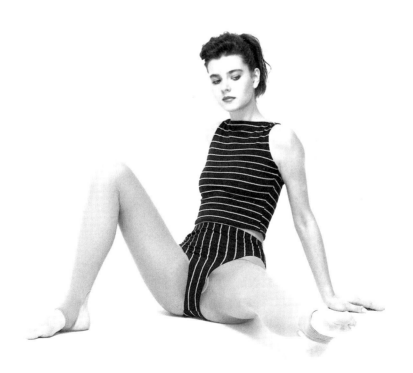

UPPER THIGH
SHAPER

---

1. • Stand straight, holding on to a support at waist level.
   • Tighten abdomen. Stand on your right leg, knee slightly bent. Raise your left knee, then kick your leg out straight in *front* of you.

• Now, pulse your leg up and down from the knee in a six-inch range.
• Continue for 30 seconds.

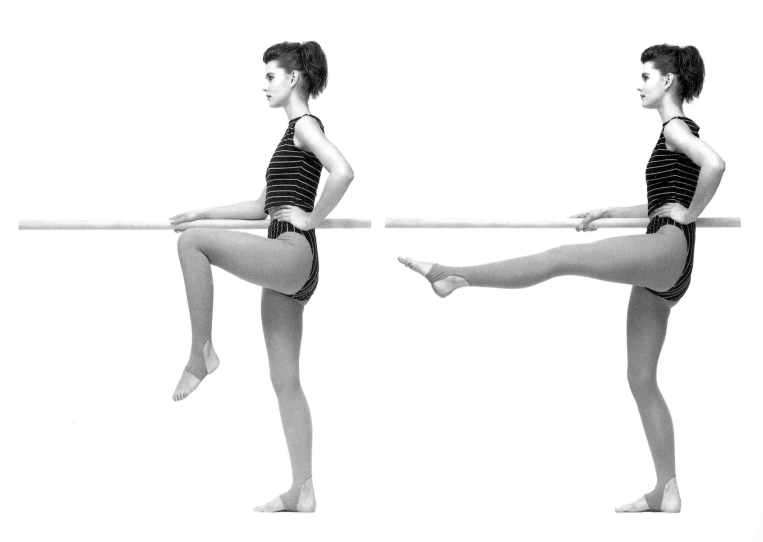

2. • Stand on right leg, knee slightly bent. Bend your left leg *back* at the knee and push it out to the side as far as possible.
 • Pulse it to the back in quick small movements for about 30 seconds.

3. • Stand on right leg, knee slightly bent. Bend left knee and kick leg to the back.
 • Push back in little pulses for about 30 seconds.
 • Repeat entire sequence with the other leg.

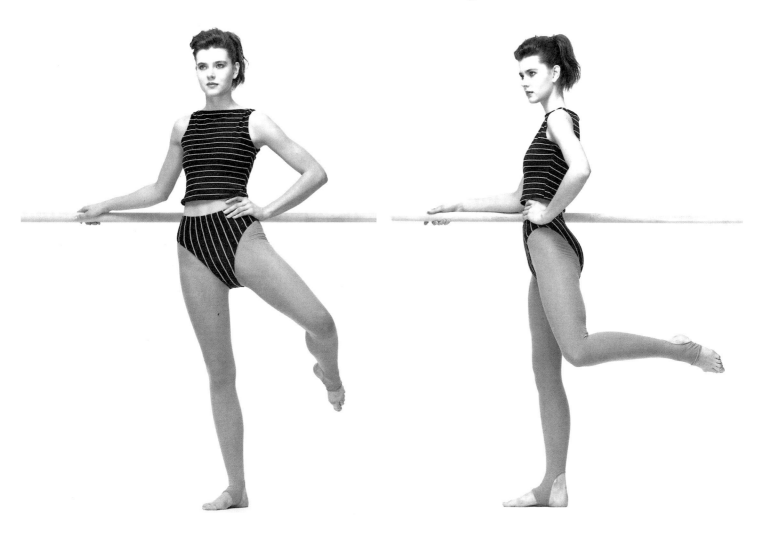

FOR THE ARMS

ANGEL
WINGS

- Stand, feet apart. Raise your elbows straight out to your sides at shoulder height, forearms dangling.
- In this position, push elbows forward, rounding your shoulders.

- Push elbows back behind you, straightening your shoulders and back.
- Repeat 20 times.

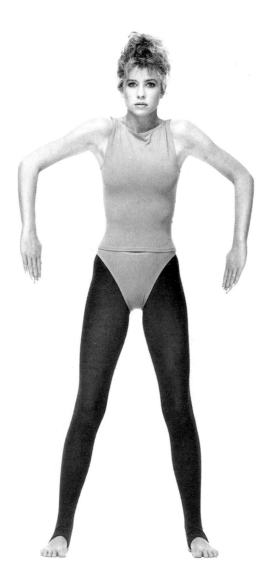

The model for the arm exercises on page 232 and pages 234–38 is Hayley Mortison.

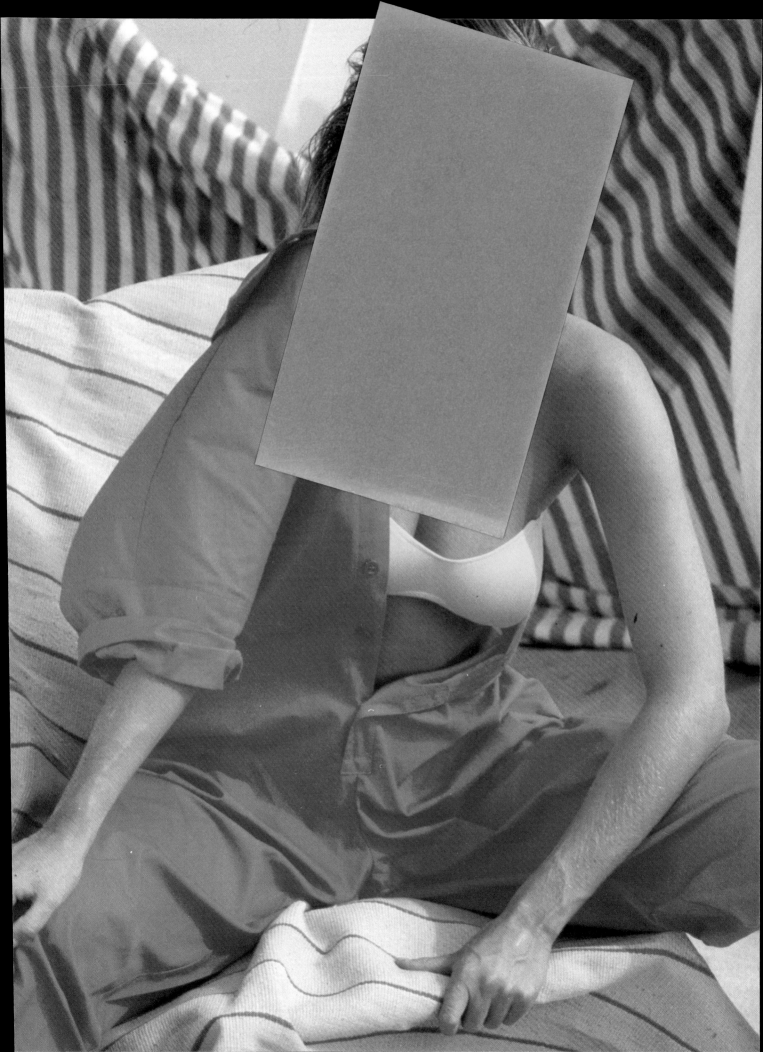

EASY
PUSHUPS

- Lie on your stomach on the floor, a flat cushion under your knees.
- Place hands, palm down, fingers forward, on the floor next to your chest.
- With your weight on your knees and hands and your back *straight*, straighten your elbows, pushing your body up.

- Bending your elbows, slowly lower your body to the floor, keeping your back straight from your knees to the top of your head.
- Repeat 20 times.

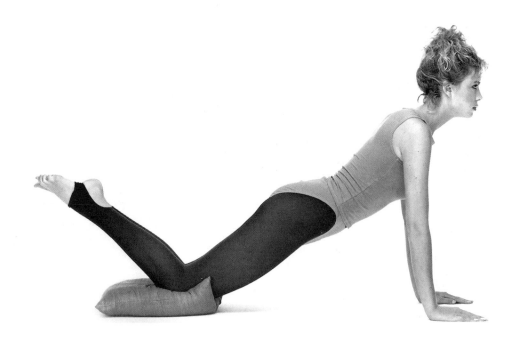

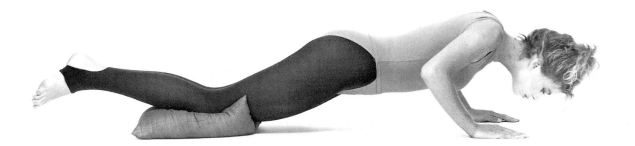

PUNCH-UP

- Stand with feet apart, pelvis tucked under and abdomen tight. Raise your elbows in front of your body slightly above shoulder level, and crook your forearms at a 90-degree angle.
- Make fists. Keeping forearms vertical and parallel, pulse alternate arms upward in quick small movements.
- Continue for about 30 seconds.

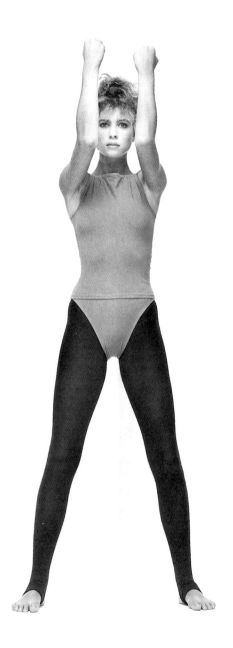

THE TENNIS
BALL

- Stand with feet apart, pelvis tucked under and abdomen tight.
- Extend arms down at your sides, hands cupped backward as though holding tennis balls.

- Pulse arms back in quick small movements, making sure to keep your shoulders down and your head up.
- Continue about 30 seconds.

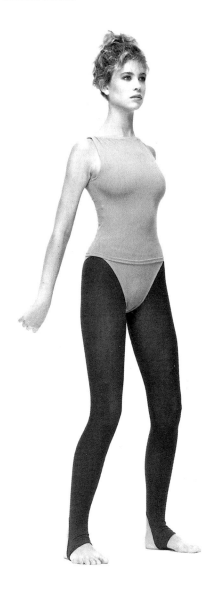
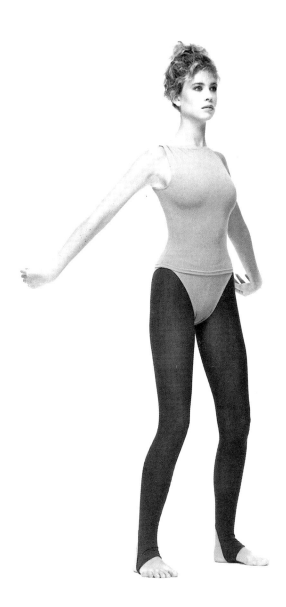

THE BIG
BIRD

- Stand with feet apart, pelvis tucked under and abdomen tight.
- Raise elbows to shoulder height and extend forearms upward at a 90-degree angle.
- Without raising shoulders, push elbows slowly forward, as though pushing against resistance, and touch them together in front of you. Hold for a count of 5.
- Return to starting position.
- Repeat 20 times.

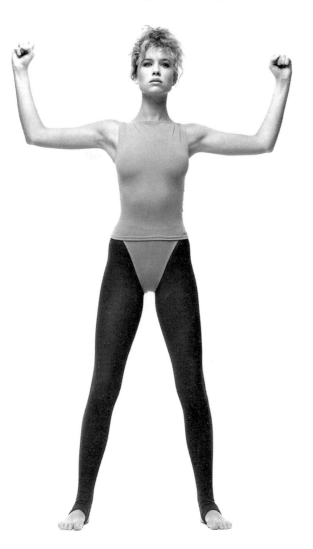
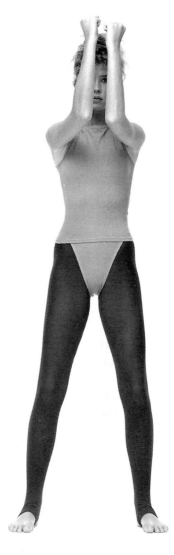

WHAT NOW?

Now that you've taken The Ford Models' Crash Course in Looking Great, don't close the books and forget all this invaluable advice from the most successful models in the business.

It isn't often the greatest models in the world share their trade secrets. Take advantage of this information to put something new into your life; you have surely found a great deal here that you can put to good use. I say it over and over again: you can be your own sort of beautiful—all you need is knowledge and the will. The last word is the real key to opening the door to a new way of living and looking. It's like deciding to plunge into a cold pool. Take a deep breath and try it. Fledgling models have to make this commitment to beauty; so do you. You would not have taken the time to read this far without having an interest in how you look. I'm sure you're now aware that you too can achieve your maximum beauty quotient with only a small investment of time.

No time? Perhaps you have a job, a family to care for and a home to run. So do models, so do I and so do so many women who always look great. They *make* the time. I know someone who constantly tells people she is so busy that she can't get all her work done. If she spent a little less time talking or thinking about how busy she is, she'd get a lot more accomplished. This same thing applies to you. Of course you are busy and pressured; that's the way of this world today. But why take only the worst of it when there's so much more there for you? Just a few minutes every day will add glamour and beauty to your life.

The Ford models and I have provided you with the tools to remake yourself. Use them to turn yourself into the beautiful woman you've always wanted to be. Start *now*.

THE FORD MODELS'
HALL OF FAME

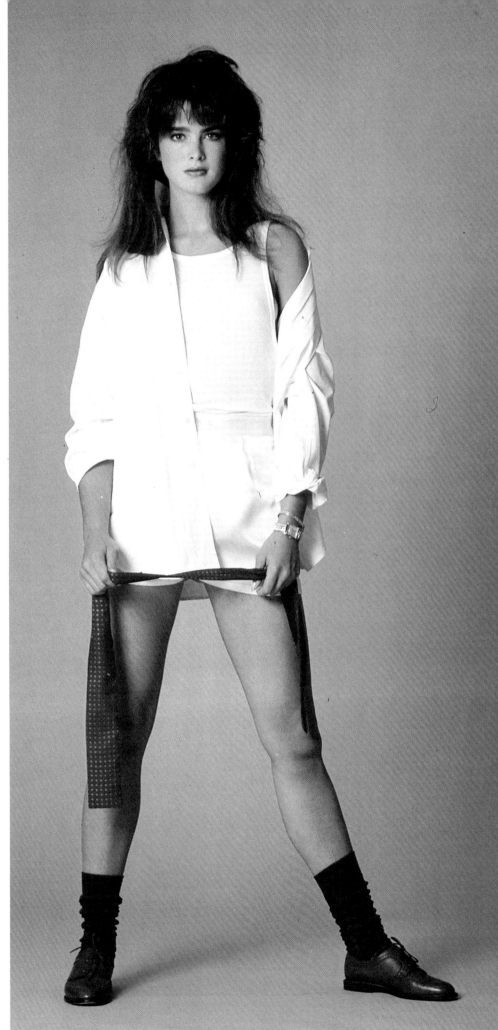

Brooke Shields. *Brooke is just as nice as she looks. At eight, she was our first child model and stayed with us until she was a teenager and her mother became her manager. Now she goes to college and leads a "normal" life, which is what she always said she was going to do.*

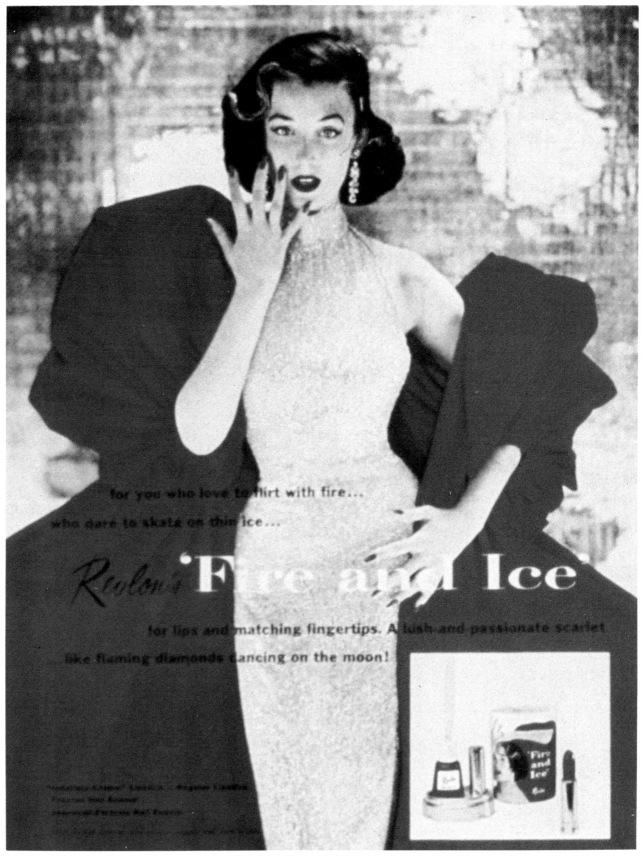

for you who love to flirt with fire...
who dare to skate on thin ice...

Revlon's 'Fire and Ice'

for lips and matching fingertips. A lush and passionate scarlet
like flaming diamonds dancing on the moon!

Dorian Leigh *was the most famous model in New York in the 1940s and probably her most famous photograph was this one for Revlon's "Fire and Ice" campaign. Always a superb cook, Dorian is a successful caterer today.*

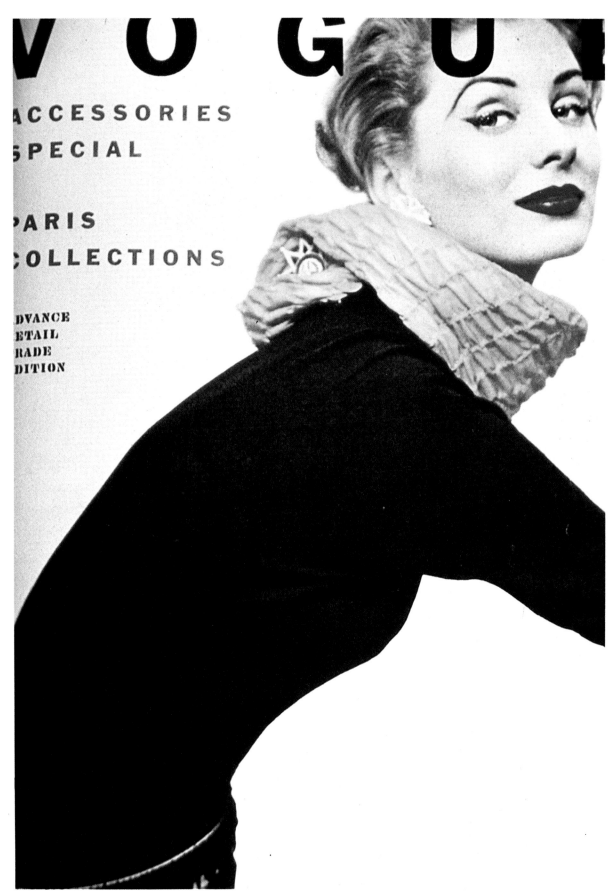

VOGUE

ACCESSORIES
SPECIAL

PARIS
COLLECTIONS

ADVANCE
RETAIL
TRADE
EDITION

Suzy Parker *is Dorian Leigh's little sister. When Dorian called us and said she'd like to work with our agency, she said we must accept her fifteen-year-old sister sight unseen. We agreed because we were eager to get Dorian, then met them both in a restaurant. Suzy was the most beautiful girl we'd ever seen. Today she's married to actor Bradford Dillman and is busy painting flowers.*

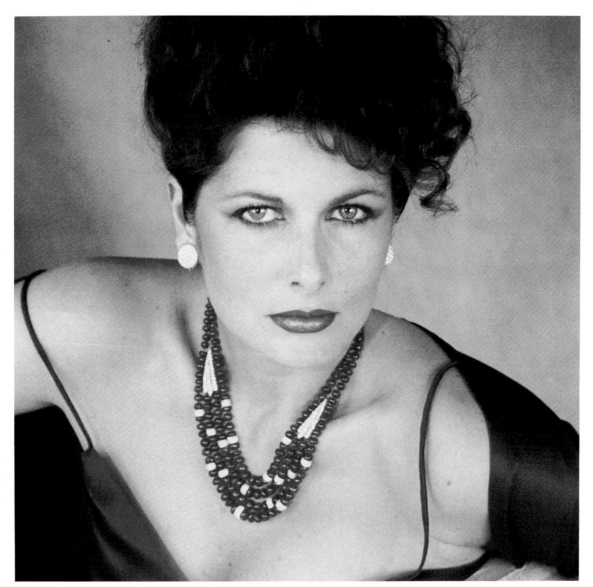

Cristina Ferrare. *She's one of the great natural beauties of the world, aside from being very intelligent and funny. Her extraordinary good humor and inner strength have seen her through many bad moments recently. It's not easy to resist her fantastic pasta dishes.*

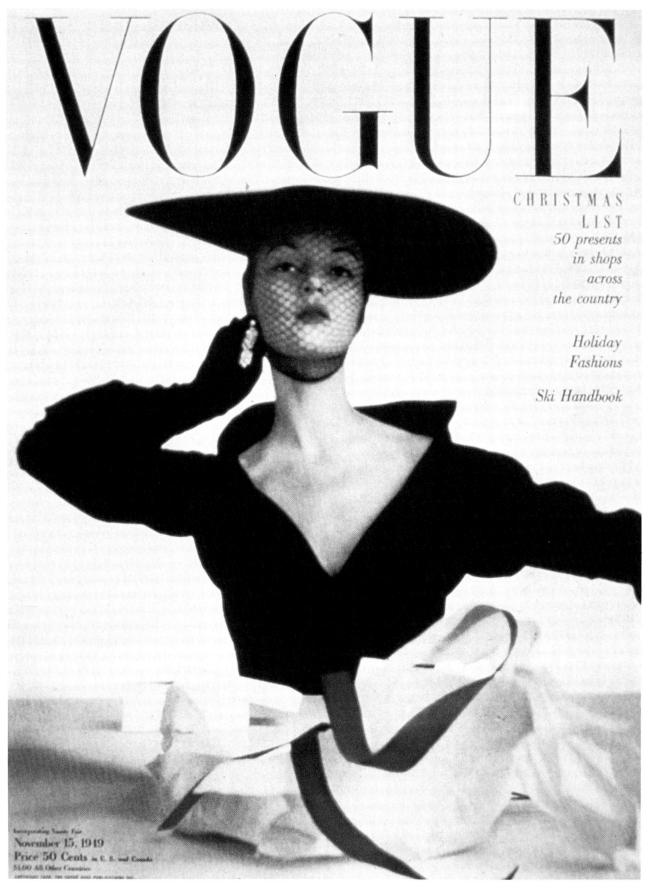

VOGUE

November 15, 1949
Price 50 Cents in U. S. and Canada
$1.00 All Other Countries

CHRISTMAS
LIST
*50 presents
in shops
across
the country*

*Holiday
Fashions*

Ski Handbook

Jean Patchett *was unique. She was to Ford Models what Babe Ruth was to the New York Yankees. She was our first great star and gave us the authority to prove ourselves as star finders. She is still a beauty and lives in California in the winter, Long Island in the summer.*

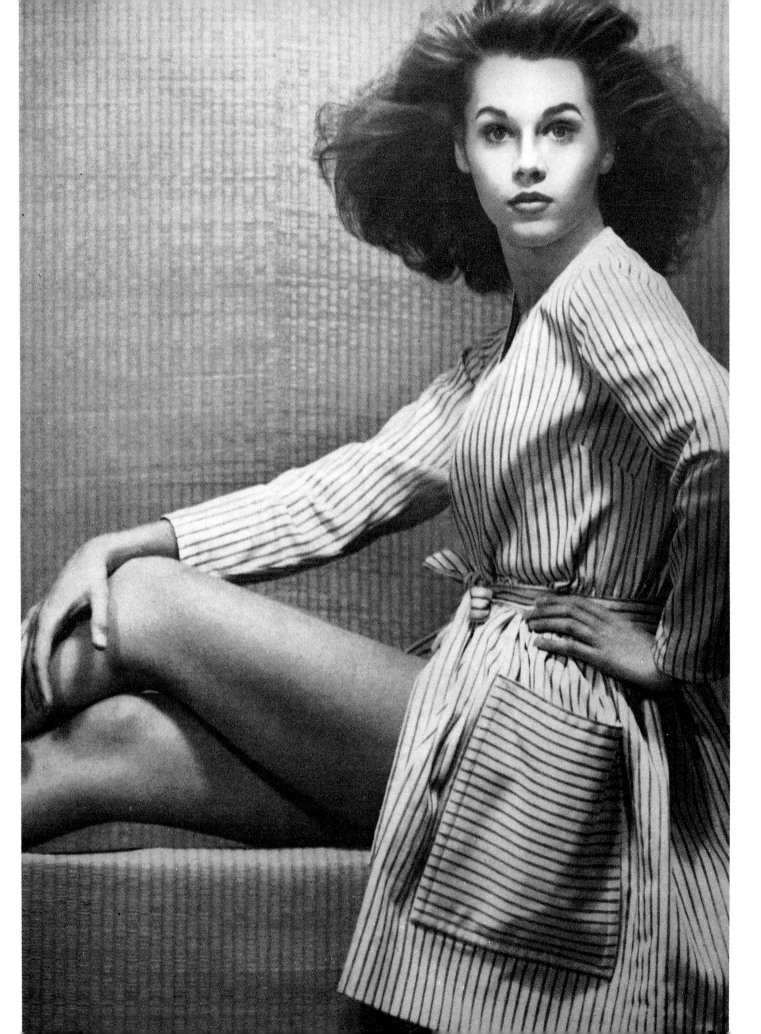

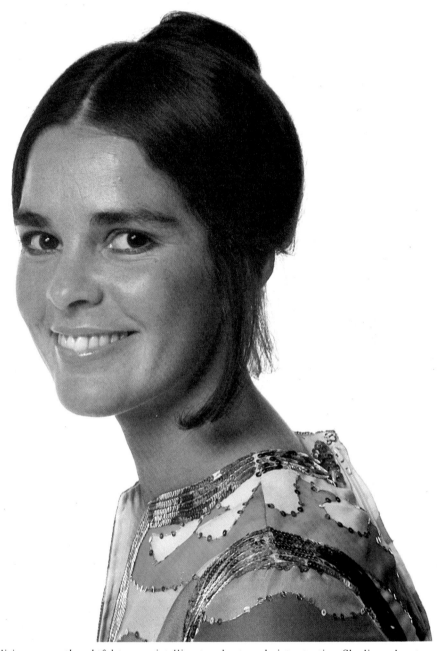

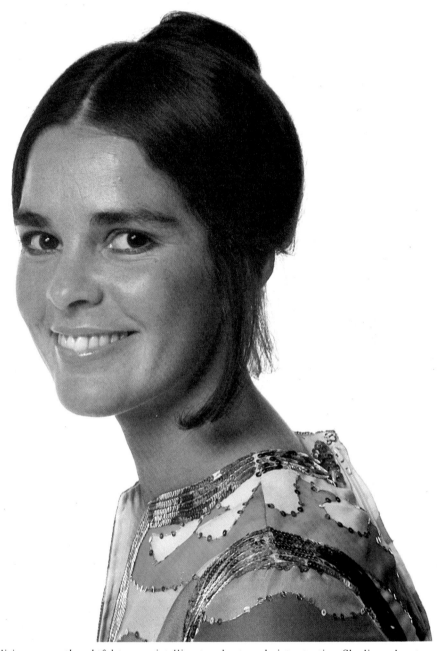 **Ali MacGraw.** *Ali is a warm thoughtful person, intelligent and extremely introspective. She lives almost a hermit life with her son Joshua and a few good friends around her. I believe it was this introspection that made her dislike modeling as much as she did. Now she's busy with a television series and decorating a new home.*

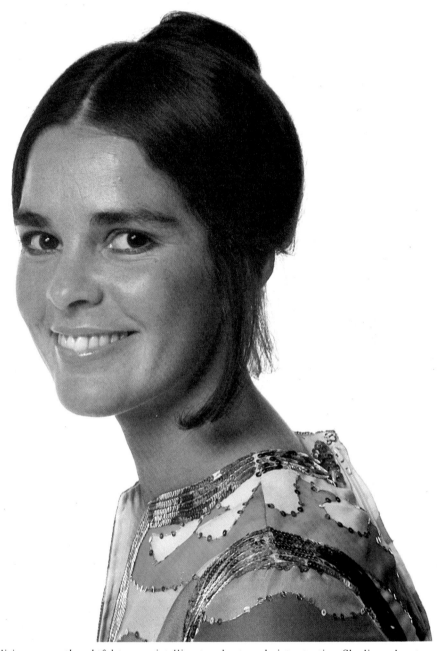 **Jane Fonda** *has always been her own person, forthright and opinionated. She was the first girl I ever knew not to wear a bra. She left us after a brief modeling career to appear in a Broadway play. After that our paths never crossed, but Jane has certainly proved that she has many talents.*

Dovima. *We found Dovima sitting on a large yacht as part of the display at the New York boat show. Although in looks she was probably the most sophisticated model we ever represented, she never lost her youthful passion for comic books and bubble gum. With her icy blue eyes and dark hair, she epitomized the remote elegance of the sixties.*

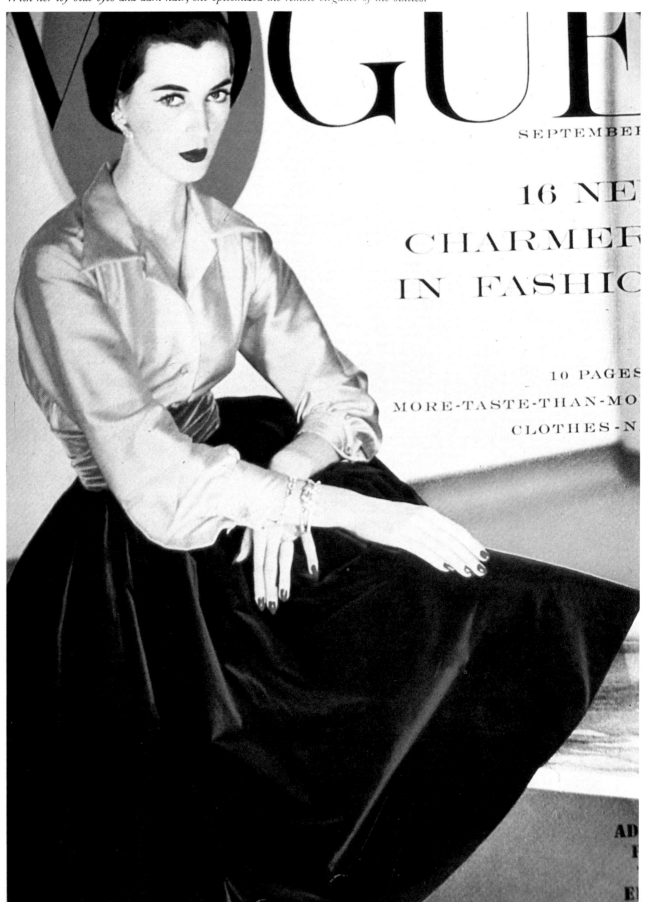

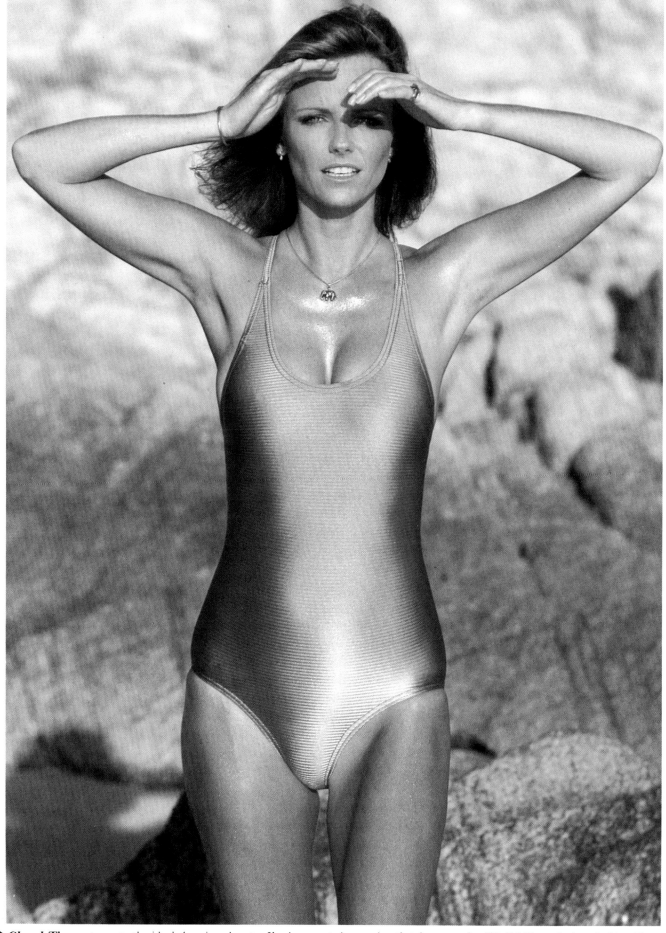

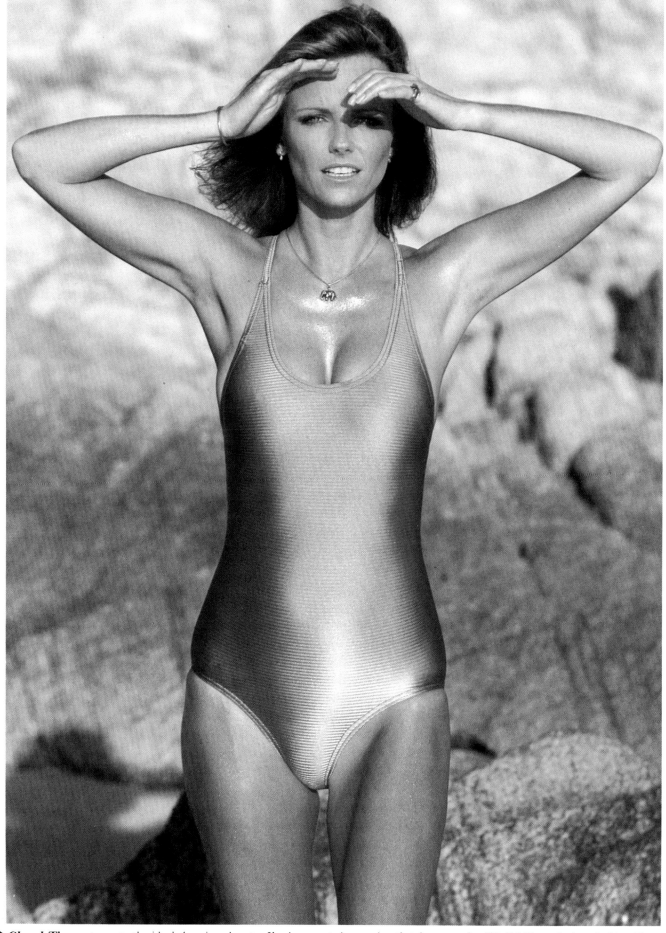 **Cheryl Tiegs** *represents the ideal American beauty. I've been quoted as saying that in some other life I'd like to be born looking like her—and it's true. She truly shines. An athletic girl from California, Cheryl is a great tennis player and works hard overseeing her line of clothes.*

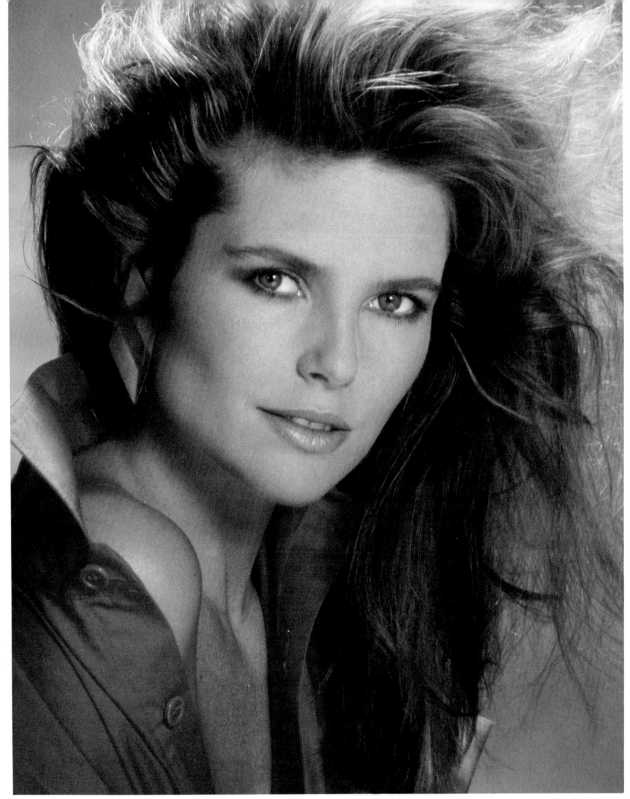

Christie Brinkley. *She's effervescent and fun, and clients love to book her because she's always so enthusiastic. Magazines with Christie on the cover outsell all others and her calendars sell just as soon as they enter the stores. So does the swimwear that carries her name.*

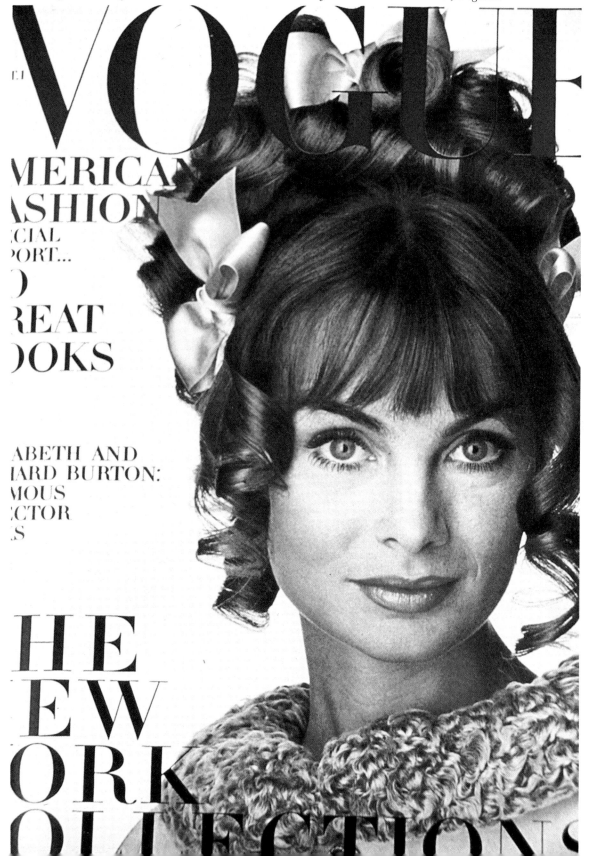

Jean Shrimpton, known as "The Shrimp," was shy and timid and had a waiflike quality. Though she was British, she looked 100 percent American. When she walked into our agency, I knew immediately that she would become a great model. Jean and her husband now run a wonderful little hotel in Penzance, England.

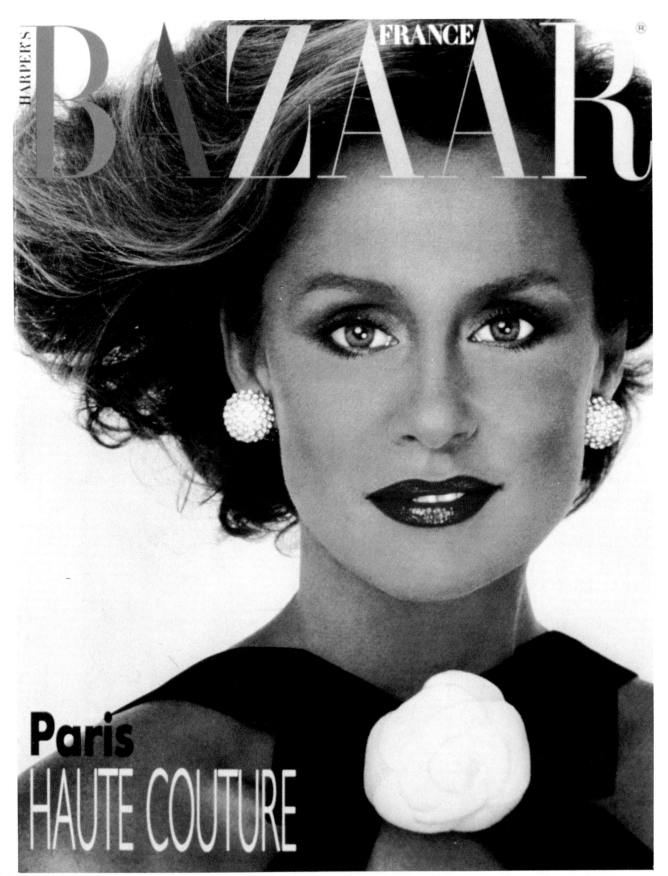

HARPER'S

BAZAAR

FRANCE ®

Paris
HAUTE COUTURE

Lauren Hutton. *She's wonderful. She probably has the best sense of humor of any model we've ever had. She's got style and self-confidence, so her one wandering eye and the space between her two front teeth don't matter. Lauren has what we call the "X Factor," the star quality the camera doesn't miss. Magazines all over the world love to use Lauren as a model between her acting assignments.*

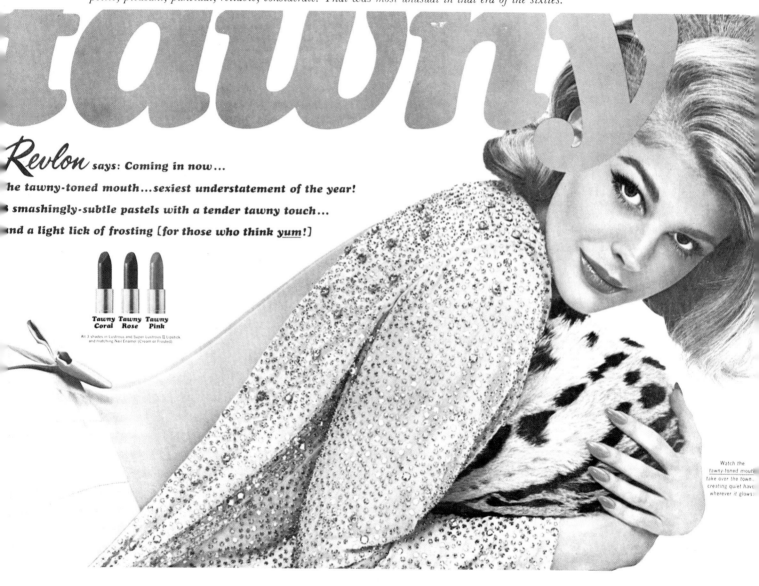

Candice Bergen. *I can truly say I never knew a nicer girl. Candy, who modeled while she was in college, was invariably polite, pleasant, punctual, reliable, considerate. That was most unusual in that era of the sixties.*

tawny

Revlon says: Coming in now...

he tawny-toned mouth...sexiest understatement of the year!

smashingly-subtle pastels with a tender tawny touch...

nd a light lick of frosting [for those who think <u>yum</u>!]

Tawny Coral **Tawny Rose** **Tawny Pink**

All 3 shades in Lustrous and Super Lustrous II Lipstick and matching Nail Enamel (Cream or Frosted)

Watch the tawny-toned mouth take over the town... creating quiet havoc wherever it glows.